Whitchurch-Stouffville Public Library

WITHDRAWN

P9-CQX-016

Whitchurch-Stouffville Public Library

Heirs of General Practice

HEIRS OF GENERAL PRACTICE

John McPhee

FARRAR STRAUS GIROUX

NEW YORK

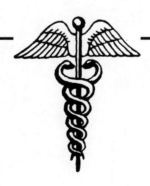

Whitchurch-Stouffville Public Library

Copyright © 1984 by John McPhee
All rights reserved
Printed in the United States of America
Published simultaneously in Canada by Collins Publishers, Toronto
This edition first published in 1986
Library of Congress Cataloging in Publication Data
McPhee, John A.
Heirs of general practice.
Originally published in the New Yorker.
1. Family medicine—United States.   2. Physicians
(General practice)—United States.   3. Medicine—Special-
ties and specialists—United States.   I. Title.
R729.5.G4M38   1986   610.69'5   84-28817
The text of this book originally appeared in The New Yorker *and was included in John McPhee's collection* Table of Contents *(1985)*

For my mother in memory of my father,
Harry R. McPhee, M.D.
1895–1984

Heirs of General Practice

When Ann Dorney was seventeen years old, she thought she might decide to become a physician. Looking for advice, she arranged an interview at a university medical center, where she was asked what subspecialty she had in mind. Had she considered neonatology? Departing in confusion, she decided instead to expand her experience as a teacher of mathematics, which, in her precocity, she already was. She had tutored other students since she was fourteen years old, and she continued to do so as an undergraduate in college. She appeared to have her future framed, but then an opportunity came along to spend a four-month work term in the office of a small-town physician. He was a general practitioner, by training and definition, but the year was 1973 and the lettering on the door had changed to "FAMILY PRACTICE." She worked in his office, went with him on hos-

pital rounds, and attended the delivery of babies. She
saw each of the other Ages of Man and an exponential
variety of cases. The math teacher began to fade again,
and she applied to medical schools—nearly a dozen in all.
Interviews were required, and she was short of funds on
which to travel. For a hundred dollars, she bought an
Ameripass, which was good on any Greyhound bus going anywhere at all within a single week. Thus, for
something like a hundred and sixty-eight hours she rode
from city to city, slept upright, checked her suitcase in
coin lockers, took off her jeans in ladies' rooms, put on a
dress and nylons, and carefully set her hair before catch-
ing a local bus to the medical school. "It was a scene,"
she says. "It was really a scene." She chose George
Washington University. As a medical freshman, when
she was asked to list her preferred specialties she wrote
"family practice" and left the rest of the space blank.
Professors attempted to dissuade her, but they were
unsuccessful.

Sue Cochran entered Radcliffe College in 1969, and
after two years felt a need to go away and develop a
sense of purpose. She went to work for a rural doctor.
Her brother, her brother's wife, her sister, and her sister's
husband were all on their way to becoming specialists
in internal medicine. Her father, a teacher at Harvard
Medical School, was a neonatologist—in her words, "a
high-tech physician." The rural doctor was her great-
aunt, who was scornful of specialists of every kind. For
decades, the aunt had looked after a large part of the
population around two mountain towns, and she passed

along to her grandniece not only a sense of what Sue Cochran calls "the psychosocial input into physical illness" but also a desire to practice medicine in a rural area and to concentrate on prevention at least as much as cure. Of her medical siblings and siblings-in-law, she says now, "They think I'm flaky." She goes on to say, "The one who's the most supportive is my father, and even he thinks I'm pretty crazy."

David Thanhauser also dropped out for a time—but, in his case, out of medical school. After graduating from Williams College, in 1969, he spent two years in medical study at Boston University before he quit, in what he now describes as "righteous adolescent anger" —angered by the world and by society in general but more specifically because he could not accept being inside what he calls "the heart of the beast of specialty medicine." In the cancer wards, for example, he felt that "technological medicine was being carried to its extreme while the feelings of people were getting no attention." In the gynecology clinic, women—many of them Hispanic or black—were given pelvic examinations before doors that kept opening and shutting. "You learn good medicine by practicing good medicine," he says. "We were learning by practicing bad medicine." In the same era, Boston revolutionaries his age were saying that while medical students were inside the hospital learning "Band-Aid medicine" a profound malaise was outside the walls. Thanhauser retreated to rural Maine, spent something under five thousand dollars (a legacy from a grandfather) to buy fifty acres of land, and, with ham-

5

mer in hand, built a small house. He thought he would give up medicine and become a teacher, but meanwhile he found work as a paramedic with generalists in Bangor. Watching these family practitioners work, he saw that they were doing an excellent job, whereas the message at Boston University had been that after people have been treated by generalists in Maine the next stop is Boston, where the damage is repaired. Before long, Thanhauser went back to medical school, but with intent to enter a family-practice residency and return to rural Maine. If such a residency had not been an option for him, his sense of conflict would not have abated and he might have abandoned medicine altogether.

Sanders Burstein, who grew up in a New York suburb, was in medical school when he made his decision, forgoing urology, oncology, nephrology, gastro-enterology to characterize his future as "family practice in a rural setting." Paul Forman made the same choice at a younger age: "I knew when I was in high school that I wanted to be a country doc." Terrence Flanagan, after finishing Harvard College, went to western Ireland for a time, and decided there that he wanted to become a doctor and practice in some remote settlement in his native Maine. After enrolling in the medical school of the University of Pennsylvania, he declared his interest in family practice. "Great," said William Penn, but almost no mention was made of the topic for the next four years. At the time of Flanagan's arrival, in 1975, the family-practice office at Penn was next door to the office of the dean; when Flanagan left, family practice was in the basement, and to get into the room you had to ask for the key. When Donna Conkling went into medicine, she had an M.A.T. in English literature from the University of Chicago. As a medical student, she was surprised one day by a resident's saying to her, "You're really smart. Why are you going into family practice?" The question seemed to her to contradict itself. Her opinion was that you had to be smart to go into family practice.

All these people—in the idiom of medical education —matched the same residency program. Specifically, they went on from medical school to complete their training at what is now called the Maine–Dartmouth Family Practice Residency, which functions principally in and close by the Kennebec Valley Medical Center, in Augusta. And so did David Jones, who knew much earlier than any of the others what he wanted to do in life. Jones is the third of five brothers. One is a nephrologist in California. Another is a cardiologist at Johns Hopkins. Their father was for many years an internist at Massachusetts General Hospital. Jones had his own idea, and he had it when he was seven. At that age, he began to say, "I am going to be a G.P. That's right, I am going to be a G.P., with a farm, a stream in my back yard, and one horse." Now, a couple of decades later, Dr. Jones has his farm, he has four horses, including an Appaloosa named Papoose, and the brooks on his land run into the Aroostook River.

While these young doctors were forming and articulating their medical bent—"to give good health care to a variety of people," and "to offer primary health care to people in a rural area"—they all had friends who were choosing things like neuropathology and otolaryngology, and were saying over their shoulders as they headed into their respected closets, "Why go into family practice? It would be so boring." Now that Jones, Dorney, Thanhauser, and the rest of them are out practicing in towns of rural Maine, they tend to remember such remarks with ironic amusement. "People said it would all be routine stuff. I never could understand that. You have an O.B., then a schizophrenic, then a well-baby check, followed by a guy with hypertension and diabetes. There is such a variety. You never know what is going to come through the door next."

Through the door next comes a woman in her upper sixties with her mother. This is not at all unusual. People over seventy bring their parents to the doctor. The daughter wears a red velvet pants suit, and the mother carries a metal cane. The mother looks about with uncomprehending interest.

"Did her eye calm down after those drops?"

"Yes, but first the trouble spread to the other eye."

"How is her appetite?"

"Good. But she won't eat fruits and vegetables. All she wants is sweets."

The dialogue between the doctor and the mother's child is like a dialogue between a pediatrician and a child's mother. Then it changes.

"I haven't been anywhere without my mother for two years."

"How long can you keep doing that?"

"As long as I have to. As long as I feel that I have to. I'll go as long as I can and then I'll quit. When my husband was around, I would get up and make a fire at five in the morning. I could go longer. Today, I don't like to get up and make a fire."

By now, it would be difficult to say which is the patient, the mother or the daughter, but the distinction is irrelevant, for both are patients here. And so, respectively, are the grandchildren and great-grandchildren of the two women. As the doctor moves a stethoscope down the great-grandmother's back, the old woman says, "I have a gizzard, maybe." On this visit, it is all she will say. She has no complaints now. Her hypochondria is gone. Her headaches are gone, and have been for three years. The doctor prescribes a cream for a facial sore. The daughter says, "She is weaker than she was. She doesn't remember five minutes. She always said she was going to live to a hundred and three, and I wouldn't put it past her."

Thirty-two-year-old male presents with warts on his penis. He is, in appearance, a woodsman—beard,

9

bluejeans, moccasins. The prescription is for podophyl-lin, an extract of the root of the mayapple. Indians were not unmindful of podophyllin. The doctor remarks in passing that some children have growths on their vocal cords that are thought to be warts. The theory is that they got them during birth, coming past the genital warts of their mothers.

Twenty-nine-year-old female presents with lesions of genital herpes. She is pregnant, and due in three weeks. Regular cultures will monitor the state of the herpes. Before labor, her doctor wants to see two con-secutive negative cultures or an obstetrician will be called in and the birth will occur by cesarean section. If labor begins while the herpes is still active, the doctors have four hours in which to complete the obstetrical surgery. If a baby is infected by herpes in a vaginal delivery, the chance is eighty per cent that it will be severely and permanently affected or will die.

Thirty-four-year-old man comes through the door with a sheath knife on his belt and a white-lettered black T-shirt that says, "MY BODY IS AN OUTLAW. IT'S WANTED ALL OVER TOWN." His leg is so full of stitches it looks like a laced boot. The doctor unlaces it.

Thirty-nine-year-old female presents with a sore throat—possibly strep, possibly viral. Her doctor knows her, and knows that the sore throat is only the precipi-tating reason for her coming in—that what she wants is general talk and counsel. Looking over her folder be-forehand, he has remarked that "any one of her problems would be enough to keep one person sick." Three weeks ago, she woke up in an ambulance, riding away from a demolished automobile. The bruises she still bears are particularly vivid because of a blood thinner that was prescribed for her when she suffered a pulmonary embolism a month before the accident. She has three children and runs a farm by herself. "The divorce becomes final on Friday," she remarks to the doctor. "Our second anniversary was yesterday." Her family could not accept her husband and made life so difficult for him he left. He is eighteen. Her first husband died of cirrhosis. Like the children, like the second husband, he was the doctor's patient, and often she has said to anyone who shows interest, "Doctor told him if he'd quit he'd live, and if he did not he'd be dead in a few months. He drank, and he died just when the doctor said he would." And now she has a question for the doctor: "Is depression an aftereffect of an accident?"

Following two well babies and a second-trimester mother, a female in her late seventies presents with a basal-cell carcinoma on the tip of her nose, growing like a small rhinoceros horn. She has a wedding to attend in two weeks, and is referred to a surgeon.

Sixty-four-year-old female presents with rashes under her arms and on her face. As before, this is merely the presenting complaint, the precipitating reason for the visit. "It's like hot coals in me," she says. "It goes right down through here, all sloomy, like a burn. It reminds me of the hospital where I had the electric shock." There are times when Oral Roberts talks with her, she confides, and her father is always with her as well. Her father is long dead. Her family has billions of dollars but not even fifty cents for her, she reports. There appears to be nothing that anyone can do to help her. Her list of problems includes but is not limited to paranoid schizophrenia, obesity, lameness, sexual dissatisfaction, hypertension, diabetes, and rash. From each regular visit, however, she seems to go away feeling a little less lost than she felt when she came in.

Smoky, wiry forty-six-year-old female presents with vague abdominal discomfort that she has mentioned before. The doctor suggests a colonoscopy, and explains that the procedure involves the insertion of a three-and-a-half-foot tube. The patient says, "I'm only five feet tall, you know."

Twelve-year-old male comes in with no complaint. He is in apparent good health, and says his mother wants him to have a physical. He removes most of his clothes. His knees are bright red from harvest work. He has made a hundred dollars in two gruelling weeks.

"What will you do with the money?" the doctor asks.

"I'm going to buy a new winter coat," he answers. "And a present for my parents."

After he leaves, the doctor says of him, "He has grown up before his time."

Next patient is the boy's mother, twenty-nine years old. She is graceful, attractive—superficially and deceptively calm. She says she has come in for a gynecological checkup, nothing more. She had a checkup not long ago. When someone comes in for a physical or a checkup, there is often a hidden agenda. "Anything troubling you today? Everything all right?" the doctor asks her.

"I work all the time," she replies. "I don't know how to relax and enjoy myself."

"Was your family like that? Your parents? Your brothers and sisters?"

"They're all nervous."

After a time, she reveals that her husband has left her, explaining that he was going away "for religious purposes." The religious purposes are that in his opinion she goes to church far too much. At home, where they live on welfare payments, it has been his habit to watch television while she almost continuously runs a vacuum cleaner. Two days ago, he returned.

"Returned?"

"He was gone three weeks. He got involved with another woman. He said the thing he got into was not meant to be. He did say that. I know we fall into traps. I told him I just don't want it to happen again. I have my church. I will not give that up. I could lean on the Lord. I may sound like a nut, but I believe in God."

The doctor lets her talk. For the moment, letting her talk is about all there is to do. The doctor sees this as his role. Part of his training has been psychiatric. Family practitioners tend to say that a gynecologist in the same situation would package the conversation, make referral to a psychiatrist, and free up the examining room for the next patient. With such remarks, family practitioners sometimes run afoul of the older specialties. In any event, this heavily distressed young woman is receiving the time she really came for. A hidden agendum is painful to the patient. Both the patient and the doctor would prefer to solve it with a pill. There is, however, no pill. "You have got to talk," the doctor tells her. "You and your husband have got to talk. Maybe he feels jealous of your church. The two of you should see a non-religious-related marriage counsellor. If you don't, you're in for trouble ahead. I worry about relationships like yours. Faith alone won't fix them." He says this, but for the most part listens.

Through the door next comes a twenty-five-year-old female who is pregnant, tall, and flourishingly good-looking, and weighs a hundred and ninety-seven pounds. The fundal height is thirty-five centimetres. Five weeks to go. The doctor listens in with a stethoscope and hears sounds of a warpath Indian drum.

Thirty-five-year-old female in a loose blouse, tight slacks, and flip-flops presents with miscellaneous pains and the information that she has not had a period in three months.

"Is there any chance that you are pregnant?"

"Jimmy had a vasectomy. Don't get me in trouble."

"Have you had intercourse with anyone but Jimmy?"

She says the doctor's first name, and adds, "Do you want to get punched out?"

He says, "Not particularly."

Her anger retreats. She tells him, "Intercourse hurts, too."

"Does it hurt when he is penetrating or when he is deep inside?"

"When he is inside. Cut three inches off and it would be all right. Cut it all off and that would be better."

Through the door comes a man who is sixty-three years old and says he is seventy-seven. The doctor asks him to say the name of the President of the United States.

The patient says, "He is an actor who used to appear with chimpanzees and was also the governor of California."

"And what is his name?"

"I don't know."

"What date is this?"

"This is the third of the month of October."

"Of what year?"

"1983."

"Fine."

"Yesterday, we had water coming down out of the skies."

"What do you call that?"

"I don't remember."

"We call it rain."

"Yeah. Rain."

The patient wears a blue polka-dot shirt. His hair is neatly combed. He is trim and kempt and appears to be some years younger than his actual age. His wife is with him. There is about them a suggestion of people who have managed their lives well and have elected early retirement.

"What did you do yesterday?" the doctor asks.

The patient says, "I went to the bank."

"On Sunday?"

"I also went to the building where they do all their business for the city."

"What do you call that?"

"I don't remember. We also went to see the Winslow Homers."

"Which ones did they have?"

"They had big ones. They had big ones this wide and this high." The patient stretches his arms wide and high.

His wife says, "He was a painter once."

The doctor says, "You seem to have trouble with your memory."

"I gave up drinking. I gave up drinking . . . drinking . . ."

"Drinking what?"

"Martinis," says the patient's wife.

The patient says, "Yes."

The doctor says, "Do you feel better?"

"Very much better. Now I drink . . . I drink . . . those little bottles they sell in the food places."

"Bottles of what?"

"Tonic," says the patient's wife.

Her husband says, "Yes. Tonic." He goes on to complain that his wife wants him to stop operating the lawn mower and driving the car.

16

The doctor says, "I'm sure that she is a good driver. I suggest that you let her drive, and grow up a little and stop complaining about it." But for pre-senile dementia, this chronic organic illness of the brain now widely known as Alzheimer's disease, there is almost nothing strictly medical that any doctor can do. There is a need to keep seeing such patients, to show them that someone professionally cares. A family doctor can do that. People who do not have a family doctor will, at dementing expense, see a neurologist instead.

David Jones' farm consists of a house, a barn, a good-sized general-utility shed, and a hundred and four acres of land, some of which is woodlot. An antique sign has been tacked up on an inside wall of the shed:

LICENSED DOCTOR

•

HEALING

•

COUNSELLING

•

HOUSE CALLS CHEERFULLY MADE

The sign dates from the era of the horse-and-sleigh, but in each of its claims and proclamations it applies to David Jones. Cheerfully, he makes house calls—gets

into his pickup, the back of which is full of farm hard-
ware and pig feed, and, with his stethoscope on the seat
beside him, goes to see a woman with severe back pain,
an old man with shingles, a woman with cancer who is
dying at home. These patients live in and near Washburn, Maine, a town with some false-front buildings and
a street so wide it vividly recalls the frontier days of the
Old East. There is a clock in the white steeple of the
First Baptist Church. The hands say eleven-forty-three
and are correct twice a day. Side streets shortly turn into
dirt roads and become the boundaries of potato fields.
Washburn has a preponderance of old and young poor.
The population is two thousand, and, often, not much is
stirring but Dr. Jones. His office is on the ground floor
of what was once a clapboard firehouse, its bell tower
still standing at one corner. Pigeons live upstairs, and
even in the walls. They make their presence heard. In
the examining rooms, they provide the white noise. They
serve the purpose Muzak serves in Scarsdale. Dr. Jones
set up his practice in 1982. In no time, word was everywhere that he would visit people's homes. "It's their
right to be seen at home if they really can't get out," he
says. "Besides that, I get to see the house, the family—
how the people live. A house call in Washburn is a town
event. The rest of the people want to know how the patient is doing. I was some sort of popular hit when I first
came up here, and I got a lot of TV coverage." The television station, in Presque Isle, which is ten miles from
Washburn and fifteen from Jones' farm, covered Dr.
Jones not only because he was some sort of popular hit

but also because he was a throwback to Eocene time. Moreover, he was a new, young, American-trained doctor in the catchment area of the Presque Isle hospital, and as such was local news. When Jones and Sanders Burstein, finishing the residency in Augusta, had shown interest in being interviewed about practicing in the Presque Isle area, the hospital offered a chartered aircraft to fetch them.

All this was happening at a time when newspapers were increasingly reporting a "doctor glut" in America, saying that too many physicians had been trained and now they were on the sidewalks looking for work. "By and large, doctors are city people" is Jones' comment. "And so are their wives. They're not willing to go out into the country. They want to eat their cake and have it, too."

In the United States, the geographic distribution of doctors is not commensurate with the spread of people generally. The ratios of doctors to various populations are, indeed, grossly atilt. By and large, doctors are city people. The percentage of doctors in big metropolitan areas is four or five times what it is in towns of fifteen to twenty-five thousand—not to mention the much lesser coverage of the small, scattered hamlets of a state like Maine. The doctor glut, if there is one, is an urban situation, and Jones seems to be right. Doctors are either unwilling or—because of the requirements of their various specialties—unable to go out into the country. Whatever the reason—from free choice to economic need—few would go as far as Jones.

If you get into your car in New York City and drive two hundred and sixty-five miles, you reach Maine. Then drive three hundred and fifty miles more and look around for Jones. His farm, by latitude, is a hundred miles farther north than Ottawa, and it is in a county that is considerably larger than the state of Connecticut. The County, as it is simply and universally referred to in Maine, has fewer than fourteen people per square mile—a statistic that owes itself to thousands of square miles of uninhabited forest. Along the eastern edge of the forest is cleared country—potato farmland—where most of the people of Aroostook County live. When they say, as they often do, that someone is from downcountry, the person could be from Mattawamkeag, sixty miles north of Bangor.

"I thought I'd have to work hard to start a practice here," Jones remarked one day about a year after his arrival. "It's been the opposite. Patients just come out of the woodwork. I'm overwhelmed. I really am." He sees them not only in Washburn but in Presque Isle as well, where thirty and sometimes forty will come through his examining rooms in a day—numbers he describes as "insane" and, whatever else they may signify, are obviously not conducive to the unhurried dialogues that are meant to knit the insights in a family practice. "I go on four hours' sleep if necessary," he said, and added, with a wistful shift of tone, "I'm a hyper individual anyway. I have to keep busy. If I slow down, I crack."

This freshly minted doctor, aged thirty-one, has a

few gray strands in his hair, which is otherwise a dark and richly shining brown, and falls symmetrically from a part in the center to cover his ears. His mustache seems medical, in that it spreads flat beyond the corners of his mouth and suggests no prognosis, positive or negative. He wears a bow tie but no white coat or any sort of jacket. In examining rooms, he has the habit of resting on his haunches while he talks to patients, one result being that he is talking up to them even if they happen to be five years old.

"Now, have a seat up here and we'll take a listen to your heart and lungs," he says to a jack-of-all-trades who is seventy-six years old and is suffering from angina. The patient goes away with a prescription for nitro-glycerin. "Old people come here once a month for reassurance," Jones remarks as he moves out of the examining room and, riffling through a family history, prepares to go into another. "The old people up here grew up in the County, and they're tremendously proud. They want to pay. Even if I say to them, 'Medicare will pay for it— you've met your deductible,' they say, 'Can't we pay you something?' You meet very proud people up here— and, with regard to health care, there is better patient compliance than you'd find in a city."

Barb Maynard is in for a check on herself and her first baby, who looks around with interest and without complaint. She is a big, strong-framed woman, who went into labor and with three pushes gave birth to a ten-pound-eleven-ounce son. Jones was much impressed.

Among his questions now is one that has to do with oats. The Joneses barter with the Maynards, baby care for oats.

A twenty-eight-year-old woman comes in with spasmodic pain in her lower right side. She suffers from adult-onset diabetes, evidently a result of excessive weight. She has dieted valiantly and has recently had a baby. Jones worries that she may have dieted too valiantly. Gallbladder disease tends to occur in women after pregnancy or after they have lost a good deal of weight.

A harvester operator comes in saying his back is killing him. Most of the year, he is a potato packer, but this is the harvest. It is the event of the Aroostook year —like June among the cherry orchards of eastern Washington. In late September, early October, schools are closed for three weeks in the County, and people from high-school age upward stand all day and into the night on the harvesters—huge crawling structures that suggest gold dredges and move about as slowly, down the long rows across the vastly cambered land at what seems like ten to the minus seven miles per hour. The people on the harvesters differentiate potatoes from glacial cobbles, to which the potatoes bear some resemblance. As the harvester operator sits on the examining table, his jeans ride up from ankle-length unlaced boots. He has a bushy beard, and his long dark-blond hair is tied behind his head. His blood pressure is a hundred and forty-four over seventy-eight. He weighs two hundred and seventy pounds.

"Do you smoke or drink?" Jones asks him.

He says, "I smoke cigarettes but mostly chew."

"You have a disadvantage," Jones says gently. "You're heavy. It aggravates back problems. It could cause a disk."

The telephone rings. The caller says, "Doc, I need an antibiotic."

"I'm sorry. I can't prescribe it over the phone."

"Doc, this is the harvest."

Jones capitulates, gives the prescription over the phone. "I have to admit I have bastardized some of my values," he says afterward. "Before I came here, I never did that. But then I had never lived in Aroostook County. If you took people from Boston or New Jersey and put them on the harvest, two out of three would die."

René Vaillancourt comes in—thirteen years old and, by law, forbidden to work on a harvester. He hand-picks. Some days ago, he cut his finger on a barrel. The skin is taut and glistens with extension. The end of the finger resembles a grape. Rainy—as his name is pronounced—is a deer hunter, and this is his trigger finger. More important to him, he is a basketball player, and the season approaches. Most important, he is missing a part of the harvest. Jones tells Rainy that for him the harvest is over, and prepares the hand for office surgery. His arm covered with green cloth, his finger presented to the scalpel, the boy asks Jones, "Will I be able to help my dad cut wood?"

"Not for a few days," says Jones.

And Rainy says, "Good."

Jones began this working day, as usual, with buttered coffee cake and a stack of bacon in the cafeteria at the Presque Isle hospital, where he spent the morning first-assisting in the operating room and making his daily rounds. He used to breakfast on three sausages and a pile of hash browns at the hospital every day, but he lightened the menu after he gained weight. Over coffee with a colleague, he talked trapping—muskrat, marten, fisher, mink—and the changeable value of pelts. When the colleague said he had picked up a beautiful mink dead on the road, Jones was thoughtful for a moment and appeared envious. He said he himself had made forty dollars last year "just on road kills," and eight hundred dollars on his fall and winter trap lines. As a boy, he trapped raccoons and muskrats along the Charles River, and on a year away from college he set up a trap line and ran it from a cabin where he lived alone in Maine. During his years in the Maine–Dartmouth residency, he set up a trap line within five miles of Augusta and brought down upon himself the scorn of other residents.

In those years, Jones also moonlighted on weekends in the County, working sixty-hour shifts in the emergency room in Caribou for twenty-five dollars an hour. It was a two-hundred-and-fifty-mile drive between Augusta and Caribou, not infrequently at twenty below zero in whiteouts with forty-mile winds, but Jones wanted the money to help pay for his envisioned farm. "In the Caribou E.R.," he says, "a lot of it was family practice: sore throats, cuts, chest pains, asthma, earaches—mundane general care. But I learned a lot, and learned to be comfortable with what I knew." Now and again, there was a chain-saw laceration, and, one weekend in three, a Code Ninety-nine. "Essentially, someone who's dead. The heart stops. You have to do your best to get it started again. The Code Ninety-nine was the most important thing I was there for—that and to keep the other doctors from having to get up in the night."

Among his patients on this September morning's rounds in the Presque Isle hospital, Staff Doctor Jones looked in on a young man—scarcely out of high school —in the intensive-care unit with aortic-root dilation. The I.C.U. has a picture window that frames the jagged silhouettes of dense black spruce and balsam fir. Moving down the corridor, Jones remarked that fourteen hours of surgery seemed to be indicated and the chance of death was one in four.

He looked in on Elizabeth Kelso, seventy-four years old. "My heart is pounding so hard," she said. "Really, it's getting me down. And I don't like the nurses."

"Blast me instead of them," Jones said. "I've got broad shoulders. You had a heart attack. Did you know that?"

Elizabeth Kelso nodded, and said to him, "I thought that's what it was."

He stopped at the beds of a chronic alcoholic with cirrhosis and a woman whose face was blotched with bruises as a result of a mysterious fall. A few hours hence, she would be given a CAT scan. Computerized axial tomography—the procedural eponym—is done by a machine that costs about a million dollars. It can discover and define tumors beyond the abilities of the X-ray.

25

A syndicate of Aroostook doctors recently bought a CAT scanner and had it fitted into a tractor-trailer. When the truck pulls up to a hospital, it is as if a 747 were docking at a gate at Kennedy. An accordion-pleated passageway distends from the hospital wall and hooks up to the trailer. Patients are CAT-scanned in the truck.

Jones had a word with Lauretta Smith, hospitalized for acute hypertension and double vision—seventy-seven years old, with Valentine-heart earrings, silver arrows through the hearts.

"They won't let me have what I see on the menu," she complained.

And Jones said, "What do you want to eat?"

"Biscuits."

"I think at your age to put you on a special diet that makes you feel bad is not a good idea. Have your biscuits. Just don't tell anybody."

"I want ice cream, too."

"You can have the ice cream."

"I don't know why the blood pressure don't stay down."

"May I have a listen to you? I want to listen to your heart."

"You knew Etta, didn't you? My sister?"

Back in the corridor, Jones said, "When people pass a certain age, the diets you impose should not be too restrictive. Eating is important, and it's one of the few recreations some older people have. You see how much she wanted a biscuit? If it keeps her cholesterol slightly elevated, what's lost? A lot is gained. I think we get hung up sometimes, running things by the book. A doctor can get too aggressive and upset the apple cart, do a lot of damage. People can be worse off than before you started doing anything."

Encountering a colleague in the hall, he was soon caught up in intense consultation. "How big are they?" he asked.

"Small."

"You're not going to eat those guys until April. They get worms. Look at their stools carefully. Clear up the worms, and pigs grow."

Jones buys piglets for twenty-five dollars, and feeds them, among other things, day-old bread, which he buys for two dollars and fifty cents a barrel. In all, he invests about a hundred and twenty dollars in a pig, and sells it to a meat market for something like three hundred. "There's easier money in doctoring," he says. "But farm money is worth eight times as much to me as money I make doctoring. Farm money is deep-rooted inside of me." Farm money and trapping money are coin of the true realm compared with the forty-five thousand dollars he was guaranteed by the hospital if he would set himself up in its catchment area—a sum, incidentally, that his earnings have greatly exceeded.

And now, in Washburn, Jones looks over the replaced fingertip of a carpenter. "When it granulates in like this, it grows slowly from the sides," he says. "I think it's going to be all right. You lost about a third of an inch."

The carpenter, Tom Dow, is a leathery man in his

sixties, who seems undisturbed. "We'll get it back," he tells Jones. "I think it will stretch out."

Joyce Sperry, seventy-one years old, has in recent times undergone a colostomy, a hysterectomy, and a vein stripping, with the result that her problem list is reduced to hypertension. As she departs for the winter in a trailer park in Florida, Jones tells her not to worry.

Hazel Campbell, seventy-seven, updates Jones on her hypertension, her edema, and her skin cancer, and bids him goodbye with a wave of a three-pronged cane.

A thirty-five-year-old man with canker sores thinks he has cuts on his tongue. Jones explains canker sores, and discovers, without surprise, that the patient loves to eat tomatoes immersed in vinegar.

Cole Chandler, nine months old and screaming, is in for a well-baby check. His mother wants to know if she should get up and care for him when he yells at night.

"Let him cry," says Jones.

After two more well babies, a mammogram, an atrial fibrillation, a chronic obstructive pulmonary problem, and a thoracic-outlet syndrome, Jones completes his day. He charges twenty dollars for an office visit, ten for a recheck. A complete physical goes for thirty-five dollars, not including lab work or electrocardiogram. "If I have to put three stitches in someone's head, that's where I can charge," he says. "I get forty-five dollars for suturing a laceration, sixty if I spend a long time. The stitches come out for free." Getting into his pickup, he drives on narrow roads through fields toward home. The sun is low. He has pigs to feed, turkeys, horses—helping his wife, Sabine, run the farm. "Doctors coin money when they do procedures," he remarks en route. "Family practice doesn't have any procedures. A urologist has cystoscopies, a gastroenterologist has gastroscopies, a dermatologist has biopsies. They can do three or four of those and make five or six hundred dollars in a single day. We get nothing when we use our time to understand the lives of our patients. Technology is rewarded in medicine, it seems to me, and not thinking."

Jones spent two high-school summers working in the Alaska Range, among people of multiple skills. The experience increased his need to be such a person, too. "I get bored doing one thing," he explains. "I admire people with ability to do different things. Within medicine, it's nice to think that I'll be taking care of the kids I deliver." His maternal grandfather and grandmother were general practitioners. They had a joint practice in Buffalo. Growing up in suburban Boston, Jones climbed trees to earn spending money—far above the ground with safety belt and chain saw, deftly amputating limbs. He became a long-distance runner, competing in Boston Marathons, and was sometimes inconvenienced when the running gave him subungual hematoma—painful pressure under the nails of his big toes. He dealt with it by heating paper clips until they glowed red, then poking them into his toenails to relieve the pressure. His surgical techniques had nowhere to go but up.

He met Sabine when he was a medical student at the University of Vermont. She was a medical-surgical technician who was born in Germany and had come to Vermont at the age of thirteen. The University of Vermont is unusual in its requirement that medical students declare a major. Jones without hesitation declared for family practice—although, by his description, "it made you a second-class citizen in some of the training."

Approaching his home, he slows down, and briefly describes his various neighbors. The dairy farmers regard him as a late sleeper. They, who get up at four-thirty, frequently call him two hours later, always with the same question—sarcastically asking, "Did I wake you?"

"I don't charge my neighbors," he says. "I don't feel right doing that." His driveway runs through woods, in which the eye threads its way to visible clearings. He pauses for a few moments after making the turn, and says, "To have a place like this was always my dream. As a physician, you can go somewhere else and make more money, but you can't live like this. You walk up on that knoll, you see Mt. Katahdin. I'd love to be a trapper in Alaska. This is my compromise."

In Sandy Burstein's office, in Mars Hill, is a bust of Julius Caesar. A quarter of the head pulls out like a piece of watermelon and exposes Caesar's brain. Burstein looks at Caesar and smiles—a subtle, rabbinical smile. The sculptor was a pharmaceutical company. The medium is plastic. The usefulness of this souvenir is in its humor, not its science.

Burstein's grandparents were emigrants from Russia, and his parents grew up in Brooklyn. In a Long Island suburb, he went to a high school so tough that he developed a way of protecting himself through what he would later call "a nonviolent approach—by avoiding conflict and befriending even the most threatening individuals." A more excellent preparation for family practice would be difficult to imagine, but in those days he had no idea that he would become a doctor, let alone a family practitioner in Mars Hill, Maine, with an office attached to a hospital of ten beds. In the words of Alexander McPhedran, the director of the Maine–Dartmouth residency, "Burstein is providing medical care that is unusual in a place as small as Mars Hill. Burstein is a very high-quality person, and the question is: Will they be able to hold him? His wife, Rowena, is from a small community near Moosehead Lake. That will help. He married well for his job."

Burstein's friend David Jones, farther up the County, describes him as "an extremely honest and thorough scientific physician" and goes on to say, "Sandy could have been good at anything—surgery, psychiatry —but he is perfect for family practice. He is low pressure, low key. He does not compromise his own values as he goes along. Seeing healthy kids, sick adults, you have to be on top of so many things. You can't sit in one little niche and know everything about it, as people in some subspecialties can."

Mars Hill, in its way, is a geographical subspecialty: a little niche in the potatoland with a catchment of people that is swollen to twenty-eight hundred by the presence of a contiguous town—Blaine, Maine. Outside Mars Hill and Blaine, Maine, are roadside vegetable stands that sell nothing but bagged potatoes. When Wilmont Kennedy, twenty years old, comes in on this September day with lobar pneumonia, Burstein knows the futility of suggesting to Kennedy that he give up the harvest and go home to bed; nor can he be much help to a thirty-six-year-old woman, who tells him she feels faint and dizzy, has lost weight and become increasingly nervous. "What's she going to do?" he says after she is gone. "It's like a no-win situation. She wants to hold her spot on the harvester." Burstein, who has a five-month-old son, declares with passion, "I hope Chaim never works the harvest."

Mars Hill, with its false fronts, is a Nevada–Wyoming Western town five miles west of Atlantic Standard Time. Its street, which seems as wide as the Champs-Elysées, is lined with angled pickups. Diesel potato trailers come pounding through. The street is also U.S. 1. Mars Hill stands in the morning shadow of a monticle of the same name—a name acquired when a British chaplain passing through here in the eighteenth century opened his Bible and began reading to his impious soldiers: "Then Paul stood in the midst of Mars' hill, and said, Ye men of Athens, I perceive that in all things ye are too superstitious. For as I passed by, and beheld your devotions, I found an altar with this inscrip-

tion, 'TO THE UNKNOWN GOD.' " Whatever its effect on
the soldiers, Paul's sermon on Areopagus has not been
forgotten in Mars Hill, Maine, where the town's other
doctor wears a cross in his lapel and has personally been
obstetricated twice. The two men—the one a newcomer,
the other in local practice twenty-one years; the one an
American, the other a Canadian; the one a residency-
trained family practitioner, the other an old-school G.P.;
the one soft-spoken, the other outspoken; the one a Jew,
the other a fundamentalist Christian—share office space.
They do not share practices, and patients sometimes
leave the one doctor for the other. That this situation
can move forward in an unincendiary way is an endorse-
ment of human nature.

Burstein is religious, too. He has sought out the
Jews of the County, a somewhat Diogenean undertaking
in a region where there is less than one Jew per hundred
square miles. Some years before Burstein's arrival, the
Aroostook Hebrew Community Center—in Presque Isle
—closed its doors, for lack of participant congregation.
Burstein travelled the County and delivered to the lapsed
families his own kind of message from Mars Hill. As a
result, the Aroostook Hebrew Community Center has
reopened. In the temporary absence of higher authority,
it is Burstein who conducts services. He is a light-framed
man with a beard, a somewhat narrow face, a benign
countenance. When a new patient sits down beside him
and answers his establishing questions, he appears to
doodle as he listens, drawing circles and squares on a
sheet of paper, connecting them in various patterns, plac-

ing an X here and there, or a number, and a word or two
as well. A circle is a female, a square is a male. A number of siblings of both sexes can be grouped within a
diamond. An X is death. A line is an interpersonal con-
nection, and if it is broken by parallel slants—//—the
people represented have been divorced. With a dotted
line he fences in current households. As his hand moves
rapidly from symbol to symbol, his attention to the patient appears to be undivided. In a few minutes of listening, he can outline something like a Russian novel, for
which this example would scarcely be a preface, with
multiple connections to come:

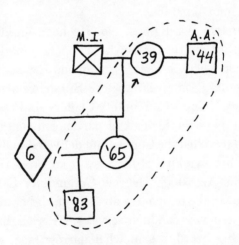

The patient (upper center) is in her middle forties,
is the mother of seven children, lost her first husband to
a myocardial infarction, and shares her present house-

hold with her alcoholic second husband (who is five years her junior) and an unmarried teen-age daughter and the daughter's baby son.

"A simple nuclear family is quite rare—and boring," Burstein says, drawing his own:

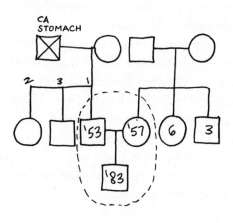

The dotted line is a house and garden on the edge of Mars Hill, and the last thing in the world Burstein really considers boring is his nuclear family. He is the oldest of three children. His wife, Rowena, is one of ten. His father died some months ago of stomach cancer, nine days after he became sick. The two were very close, and the son will not soon recover. His sense of family—beginning with his own and extending to anyone's—appears to be what caused him to choose this form of practice over all else in medicine. David Jones has said of him, "He deeply believes that you can deliver better medical care by taking an interest in a whole family. He is clear about his goals."

A semantic distinction has been drawn between family practice and family medicine, the one being a form of medical service, the other being an academic discipline. Family medicine is an approach to practice, and is constructed around the unquantifiable idea that a doctor who treats your grandmother, your father, your niece, and your daughter will be more adroit in treating you. After Oberlin College, Burstein went to the medical school of Case Western Reserve University, where he studied under Dr. Jack Medalie, who had compiled a textbook called "Family Medicine" and written much of it as well. Also at Case, Burstein learned the graphic form of shorthand known to doctors as genograms.

From a folder he removes what to him represents an ideal collection of patients:

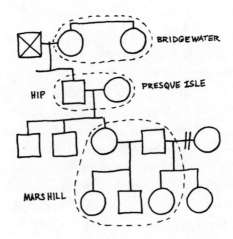

There are four generations—thirteen living people, and nearly all of them are his patients: the old sisters, who live together in Bridgewater; the grandchildren and great-grandchildren, in Mars Hill; the grandfather from Presque Isle, with the trouble in his hip.

Burstein's telephone rings. The caller is Margaret Cunniff:

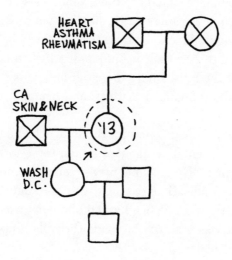

She is not a regular complainer, and she wants him. He gets into his car and goes. She lives out by Adelman's potato storage. Tons of firewood lie by her house un-stacked. She is shaking, shivering, and has had what she calls "a puking spell." She is graceful and gracious despite her considerable discomfort. Burstein gives her an antiemetic. She seems not to notice his invading needle. She has chronic rheumatoid arthritis, next to which this virus is a passing irritation. To be old, it helps to be tough, and she has lots of help.

Back in the office, Richard Hatfield is waiting, a burly man of forty-five with a ruddy face and a red beard. He wears laced twelve-inch boots, and dark-green work clothes with sleeves rolled. Some years ago, he suffered a myocardial infarction. Nonetheless, he delivers ninety-two newspapers daily, starting out at 2:30 A.M., now and again in temperatures around thirty below zero. "If I had a three-speed, I could do it a little quicker," he says. "On the hills, I have to get off and walk." Hatfield worries about financial matters, and brings his worries to Burstein.

A new patient comes in. Burstein asks him who his doctor has been. The name of a man some towns away is mentioned. "He gave me fifty green pills and he gave me fifty red pills. The red ones were for stomach. They cleared it right up. When I asked him what was in them, he said it was a secret, he made the pills himself. He's wealthy, I believe."

"So I understand."

"Doctor I went to, used to be in Caribou, he closed up and went back to India. And that Korean, the only reason he had to leave was his skin was yellow and people here didn't believe in it. The last time I went to a doctor, I asked him, 'Are you going to take blood or give it?' He said, 'Take it, naturally.' And I said, 'No, you're not,' and I walked out, and I ain't seen a doctor since. Now I'm trying you."

Burstein gives no indication that he is flattered.

Wilmont Kennedy, unable to continue on the harvest, comes back to Burstein's office. Clutched in the patient's hand is a can of Pepsi-Cola. He is running a fever. His heart is beating a hundred and seventy times a minute in atrial fibrillation. There is a loud murmur. An X-ray picture made as a result of his previous visit shows a heart of unusual shape, with a narrow pedicle and an over-all size that borders on the abnormal. "Stale Pepsi will take care of this," he tells Burstein. "It always does. I'll feel better after I've had this soda, I know I will. I'm having a six-pack attack."

Burstein has alternative ideas. He calls the intensive-care unit at the Presque Isle hospital, fifteen miles away. "Do you have any beds up there? Good. You have a patient." He calls a cardiologist. He mentions congenital cardiac anomaly, possible infection in a heart valve. At the very least, the patient must be cardioverted to quell the fibrillation. Burstein calls an ambulance. When it arrives, Wilmont Kennedy is placed on a rolling stretcher, his long blond hair cascading off the sides toward the floor. He rests the Pepsi on his chest. As the wheels move and his journey begins, he says, "This is Class One."

When Kennedy is gone, Burstein sits contemplatively beside the bust of Caesar. After a time, he says, "What is most interesting in family practice is not what

the problem is but what motivates people to seek help
for it. Something in the family, a hidden factor, will
make the mundane interesting. If you are a cardiologist,
you know your patient has a heart problem when the
patient comes through the door. When someone comes
to a family doctor, the doctor is starting from scratch.
There can be underlying components, psychological or
social. The purpose is to help people in a deep and per-
sonal way. I was attracted from the beginning to the
variety of things family doctors do. And I liked the people I saw going into family practice. I'm not always sure
it was the right choice. Life might be easier if I were a
respected urologist."

B urstein goes to the emergency room because
Tim Brewer has fallen off the monkey bars at the Fort
Street School. Tim is seven, wears corduroy jeans and
running shoes, and has a gash in the top of his head. A
grandmother is present. Burstein works without hurry,
conversing with Tim, whose fortitude deserves the com-
pliments he receives. There are multiple pricks of lido-
caine, splashes of hydrogen peroxide, followed by
syringed water. The lad's chin is high. He sits rigidly
upright. Burstein ties stitches like dry flies. When he is
done, Barbara Smith, R.N., leans forward and carefully
combs Tim's bright-blond hair.

The scene strongly brings to mind a stack of magazines tied up with string in an attic. It strongly brings to mind that medical superman of yesteryear, the old doc on the cover of *The Saturday Evening Post* with his stethoscope planted on the chest of a child's doll, the old doc who rode from house to house through deep snows with his black bag beside him and his roan gelding pulling the sleigh, the old doc who did appendectomies on the kitchen table, the old doc who worked nine days a week and rested on the tenth. If the social status of a urologist, a nephrologist, a gastroenterologist can send a wistful moment through the thoughts of a family practitioner, that is as nothing compared with this hovering ghost, this image afloat above the family practitioner's head: Superdoc, the Great American G.P., omniscient, ubiquitous. Who will ever forget his snowshoeing through the Blizzard of '88 to set Increase Flintcotton's broken leg? Never mind that despite old Superdoc's gruelling schedule he somehow had time to sit for Norman Rockwell while the artist did one portrait after another, from this angle and that. Never mind that old Superdoc saw three, and sometimes as many as five, patients a day. Never mind that in the course of his long career he saw so little medicine that his scientific knowledge steadily declined from new to nil. All of that is gone with the blizzards; and what is left behind is his mythic standard.

The age of medical technology began to pick up great momentum around the time of the First World War, and with it consequentially came the age of specialization. Beforehand, almost all doctors were general practitioners. As specialists and subspecialists began to develop, the number of G.P.s went into a fifty-year decline, and by the middle nineteen-sixties G.P.s were becoming scarce, if not approaching extinction. To the layman—the neighbor, the patient—who looked back upon the old superhuman doctor with admiration, imagination, exaggeration, and nostalgia, it seemed that a form of giant had disappeared. It also seemed that, as in most human pursuits, when giants shuffle off the coil they are replaced by committees. Gynecologist, urologist, nephrologist, immunologist, pediatric oncologist, neuro-ophthalmologist, psychopharmacologist, coronary angiographist—through time the specialists had subdivided and subsubdivided, advancing and serving technology. The positive effects of this history—and of the research that created new machines and new procedures and new subspecialties to accompany them—were dramatic and considerable. In no way were they diminished by the concomitant eventuality that some effects were negative.

The committee—which seldom, if ever, met—took on the numbers of a crowd. No one seemed to be in charge. The patient, in the process, was not so much quartered as diced. People were being passed like bucks —or so it seemed to them—from doctor to doctor. Even such a traditionally one-on-one event as the "complete physical" might be subdivided, as internists who did not do pelvic or rectal examinations sent their patients on to gynecologists, proctologists, or urologists. Most people could not say that they had a regular doctor. Most people did not have access to a doctor who had the time—or maybe the inclination—not only to deal with them when they were sick but also to help keep them from getting sick in the first place. There was such an absence of doctors with varied general training that someone in, say, a small Maine town would have to travel large distances just to do something as natural as have a baby. For many people, the fees of specialists were prohibitive. People wanted health care. They wanted it locally, and they wanted it at a price they could afford. Also, they wanted something more on the other side of the Rx pad than a dispenser of penicillin. In growing numbers, they felt confused and used. Was there a doctor in the house who could still regard a patient as a person rather than a disease?

To many young doctors, a clearly defined niche of technical competence seemed preferable to the complexity of general practice. To varying extents, specialists could retreat into their specialties. As the medical technocracy grew, it reproduced itself, by contemplating the pool of medical students and choosing its own kind. In their concentration on a single topic, most doctors seemed more than willing to risk losing touch with medicine as a whole. The old doc of the magazine cover —magician, counsellor, metaphysician—had been replaced by technicians with machines and clipboards.

As specialization increased and the old doctors faded away, a patient, when need came, often had no idea what to do to get into the system. Over time, the hospital emergency department became the portal of entry—in various ways a forbidding prospect. Moreover, the price of entry was high. A hospital emergency room (known in some parts of Maine as "the Band-Aid station") has to be staffed to take care of everything from automobile accidents to aneurysms, myocardial infarctions to gunshot wounds, and therefore the cost of a walk-in visit for a sore throat or an enigmatic pain might be four times what the cost would be for an office visit to a general, nonexistent practitioner. So people stayed home. If they had pneumonia, for example, and might have been treated effectively while they were moderately sick, they tended to let it go, and too often they developed abscesses that required surgical draining and in some cases caused death. Getting into the system early was important, but if it meant going to the emergency room for many dollars, a person might not go. A reaction was coming. And by the middle nineteen-sixties it was overdue.

"It had to come, because we weren't taking care of people's little needs," an internist candidly, if somewhat sardonically, admits. "You can't blame the people, because they weren't getting good service. They were getting specialists and subspecialists, and not enough hand-holding. That's a legitimate role for a doctor to play. It should be the primary role."

The reaction became known as the family-practice movement. Its aim was to shift some of the emphasis in medicine, to give refreshed importance to generalism; and it arose, of course, at a time when many people had come to distrust the pervasion of technology in every field from high-energy physics to superfast foods, and to look upon the dehumanization of medicine (a phrase much in vogue) as just one of a great number of unfortunate results. Thus, the family-practice movement drew stimulus not only from within the medical profession, where it was controversial and was not infrequently damned, but also from sources as broad as the society itself. While environmentalists were coming into their moment of sunlight, and pantheons everywhere were sprouting new gods, old Superdoc was invited to return to medicine. To bring him back (in modern form), the American Board of Family Practice was conceived and established.

Inevitably, the federal government had entered the conversation. In the years since the Second World War, very large sums of national money had been spent on medical research—notably in assaults on heart disease, cancer, and strokes—and the government was not satisfied that the useful results of the research were being properly spread about, especially to places where populations were thin. There had been studies and reports on medical education and manpower distribution, and regional medical programs had been set up to help relieve deficiencies. Nothing would provide such relief more effectively than a large new influx of general physicians. There had been nineteen specialties in medicine. In 1969, family practice became the twentieth.

The news was particularly welcome in a state like Maine, which was largely rural (where it was not wild) and did not have a medical school. There had been one, at Bowdoin College, but it closed its doors in 1921, and since then Maine had parsimoniously got along, eating its apple a day—and shrewdly depending on its beauty, among other things, to attract doctors from elsewhere. This worked tolerably well but not perfectly. In unattractive places where there was nothing much to do but swat blackflies, doctors were particularly scarce. In Maine cities and large towns, as everywhere in the nation, the number of specialists was grossly disproportionate to the number of doctors engaged exclusively in primary health care. Now, however, with the new specialty of family practice, there might be a way to redress these needs. A family-practice residency—inclining, as it would, to outpatient care—could be set up at a community hospital and did not have to be part of a major urban medical center. In some ways, a community hospital would actually be a preferable setting. Statistically, doctors tend to go into practice near their residencies. This fact had made its way to Maine. Maine might not have a medical school, but if Maine were to set up a family-practice residency somewhere reasonably distant from all its borders Maine could virtually rely upon a majority of the product doctors to spread out into and stay forever in Maine.

The Central Maine Family Practice Residency, as it was first called, was established in 1973, at the Kennebec Valley Medical Center, in Augusta, the state capital. Over the years, its rotations have involved other hospitals in the region— most notably the Mid-Maine Medical Center, in Waterville—always with the advantage to the young doctors that they are the only residents there. They have the hospital-staff doctors' undivided teaching attention, and do not have to stand by, as family-practice residents in large urban medical centers often do, while specialists clone themselves—while, for example, cardiologists concentrate on teaching residents who are future cardiologists. Simultaneously, the family-practice residents have a considerable uplifting effect on the community hospital. It is a datum that cannot be measured, but the quality of care in the Kennebec Valley Medical Center is in all probability superior to what it would be in the absence of the residency, because the hospital's staff doctors must, as teachers, be especially current on the matters they teach. Following the Kennebec Valley example, Lewiston, Bangor, and Portland established family-practice residencies, and spread the values of the teaching hospital in Maine. In 1979, Dartmouth Medical School, not far away, in New Hampshire, affiliated its family-practice department with the Augusta residency, making a joint declaration of a mutual goal: "To produce family physicians who are concerned with, and thoroughly schooled in, the effective delivery of comprehensive medical care in rural communities."

Now, in the middle nineteen-eighties, there are about seven thousand young doctors in family-practice residencies around the United States. Family practice has become, after internal medicine and surgery, the third most popular choice in specialties among graduating seniors in American medical schools. Some disparaging doctors seem to enjoy suggesting that family practitioners are at the low end of the totem of medical I.Q., but in point of fact that distinction belongs to the family practitioner to no greater extent than it does to the disparaging doctors. Competition for the Maine–Dartmouth residency is especially stiff. Annually, about a hundred people apply for six positions—after travelling north and seeing for themselves that, as one of them has put it, "you don't have to choose between good medicine and living in Maine." Their training takes place not only in hospitals but also in an office setting, in a building of their own in Augusta called the Family Medicine Institute, where the residents—usually about eighteen in all—see twenty-two thousand patients a year. Half the residents are women. Asked why the number is so large, when the ratio of men to women in American medical schools is at present three to one, Maine–Dartmouth's director, Dr. Alexander McPhedran, says, "Because we worked at it."

As the number of doctors going into family practice has risen, the number of doctors going into psychiatry has declined. This to some extent suggests the sort of person who is attracted to family practice—suggests where, on the human spectrum, the seven thousand residents have come from. Dr. H. Alan Hume picks up this theme: "Family practice does not appeal to many types of people; family practice does not appeal, for example, to the impatient egotists who are attracted to surgery." Hume is a general surgeon. He is also a spontaneous conversationalist, who practices in Waterville, Maine, and has taught for many years on the Maine–Dartmouth faculty. He continues, "Family practice is unlikely to attract the sort of person who will one day be saying, 'Don't bother me with details, I've already made up my

mind, let's cut.' Or 'If you can't cut it out, it isn't worth
treating.' Or 'When somebody comes in with a rigid
abdomen, high white count, fever, shock, all I care about
is that I put the incision in the right place. It's em-
barrassing to make two.' The sort of people who go into
neurology are also not likely to choose family practice.
Neurologists are known for studying things until hell
freezes over, because they don't have to make decisions.
People who like oncology like to—in a leisurely way—
deal with malignant tumors with chemotherapy. Internists enjoy the challenge of a diagnostic problem. A patient has ill-defined pain: What is it? How can I find a
right answer with two tests instead of ten? People who
go into family practice experience real joy in dealing
with people, and have a sense of wanting to be generalists. They also have a tremendous sense of obligation to
community, which is much less true of surgeons and
internists. You'll find the family practitioners out there
on the athletic fields in the afternoons as school-sports
doctors. You'll find them running things at the P.T.A.
They're into the community, and they're willing to have
lesser incomes."

Family practitioners have been described by other
doctors as "people people—not in medicine for the technology."

"They are more conscious of social purpose than
other physicians."

"They are interested in the biology of medicine,
yes, but they are equally interested in what people's lives
are like—in how people relate to one another in a family."

The old general practitioners, after finishing medical school, went through one-year rotating internships and then out into the community. As their numbers dwindled through time, so did their status, because they came to be regarded as undertrained. With the creation of the American Board of Family Practice, it was decided that the new "specialists" would not only undertake full three-year residencies but also be required to sit for reexamination every seven years for the rest of their professional lives—a requirement unique in the profession. Not without a dash of oxymoron, the Accreditation Council for Graduate Medical Education defined family practice as "a comprehensive specialty." In amplification, the council mentioned "responsibility for the total health care of the individual and family," and went on to say that all family practitioners must be adequately versed in gerontology, including "preventive aspects of health care, the physiological and psychological changes of senescence, the social-cultural . . . nutritional and pathological (acute and chronic) entities of aging"; in psychiatry, including psychotherapy, psychopharmacology, psychiatric counselling, mental illness, alcoholism, and other substance abuse; in internal medicine, including cardiology, endocrinology, pulmonary diseases, hematology, oncology, gastroenterology, infectious disease, rheumatology, nephrology, immunology, and neurology; in dermatology; in pediatrics; in obstetrics and gynecology, including "skills in marriage counseling, sex education, human sexuality, and family planning"; in surgery, to the extent of being able to diagnose and

manage surgical emergencies, make "appropriate and
timely referral," give "proper advice, explanation, and
emotional support to the patients and their families,"
give pre-operative and post-operative care, and acquire
enough understanding of basic surgical principles,
asepsis, and the handling of tissue to qualify as a first
assistant for a surgeon in the operating room; in emergency medicine, including advanced cardiac life support,
airway insertion, chest-tube insertion, and hemostasis;
in orthopedics, ophthalmology, otolaryngology, and
urology; and in diagnostic imaging, including the in-
terpretation of radiographic film. The old term "G.P."
had been given a semantic sandblast. The new board-
certified practitioners were being called specialists to
legitimize the fact that they were not.

Fred Schmidt, thirty-three years old, is, among
other things, a woodcutter, who gets forty-six dollars a
cord, and works alone.

"Smoke?"

"I quit four years ago."

"Why did you quit?"

"The time had come."

Schmidt is in for a routine physical—Lovejoy
Health Center, Albion, Maine. A muscular man with
curly hair and a woodsman's ample mustache, he is so
healthy that Paul Forman, the examining doctor, won-

ders if he has a hidden agenda. As they converse, however, there is no hint of trouble, and Forman begins to feel oddly guilty for not giving Schmidt his money's worth. Forman feels as if he is purloining half a cord of wood from this well-kept human landscape. Rummaging, he asks Schmidt if he uses hearing protection when he operates his chain saw. Schmidt says no. Forman's conscience is saved. He will give Schmidt some preventive medicine—sawed, split, and stacked.

Old-time pilots in open cockpits used to get something called aviator's notch, Forman says, and he draws on an audiogram pad a graph that shows a precipitous loss of hearing high in the frequency range of the engine of a Jenny or a Spad. The loss appears on the graph as a V-shaped notch. "The airplane engines gradually destroyed the ear's ability to pick up any sound in those frequencies," Forman continues. "If you don't protect your ears, you are in danger of getting aviator's notch from your chain saw. We see similar things with rock and roll." Partial deafness is only the beginning. In the literature on amplified sound, there appears this sentence: "Loud noise causes blood vessels to constrict, the skin to pale, muscles to tense, and the adrenal hormone to be injected into the bloodstream; thus, the heart and nervous system of the individual are profoundly affected; animals, forced to listen to noise, become sullen, unresponsive, erratic, or violent."

Has Schmidt ever heard of Iowa ear? The farmer on his tractor looks over his right shoulder, watching his planter or plow and sighting back down the row. This aims his left ear toward the tractor's engine. Iowa ear, always the left, is aviator's notch, grounded.

Schmidt hears all this amiably, perhaps even gratefully, giving no sign that he has developed a notch of his own with regard to doctors.

Forman changes the subject. He asks if Schmidt's wife, Terry, is having contractions.

"Not yet."

Forman will deliver this imminent baby. He also looks after the Schmidts' existing child. Half a dozen years ago, before Forman and his partner, Forrest West, arrived in Albion, the Lovejoy Health Center was an overgrown field. "Before the clinic was here, I didn't have a doctor," Schmidt remarks. "When I needed a tetanus shot, I drove twenty miles to the Band-Aid station. They said come back tomorrow. I went to a doctor's office somewhere. They said forget it, you're not a regular customer."

Forrest West, in an adjacent examining room, talks with Seth Fuller, a farmer, born in 1904. Fuller is West's neighbor. Fuller remembers when West and Forman first came into the area and went to potluck suppers and casserole dinners, meeting people and asking about plans for a health center—in effect, applying to be its doctors. Six communities—China, Albion, Unity, Palermo, Thorndike, and Troy, which are separated by dairyland and forested hills—had been identified by the federal government as grossly underserved, and money had been raised locally for a modest wooden structure. Forman and West were, in Forman's words, on "the hippie wavelength," but their credentials were even longer than their hair. They were strongly recommended by the residency in Augusta. Fuller and the others voted them in.

Fuller's wife, Gladys, is in the exam room, too. She was West's first myocardial infarction in Albion. She has recovered long since. It is her husband who has now come in with the presenting complaint. He can describe it only as "a gradual weakening." He says he lies on the couch at home sleeping and when he wakes up is not interested in stirring. He has let the farm become inactive. He is trim, short, with a wiry frame and alert eyes —obviously, in his demeanor if not his present manner, a hardworking, life-loving man. His hair is steel gray and cut short—like his accent, which is pure Maine. "I suppose I could feel worse, but I don't know that it would make much difference," he says. He has had recent X-rays that looked normal, and a blood test as well. "There's an end to that dragging down," he tells West. "I can't go on losing weight forever." He weighs a hundred pounds. Two years ago, he weighed a hundred and four. He removes his shirt. His biceps suggest considerable strength despite his frailty. West listens to his lungs and heart. What could be Seth Fuller's difficulty? An occult malignancy? Stomach not absorbing vitamins? He had a partial gastrectomy, West remembers, but that was some time ago. He tells Fuller that he would like to admit him to the Mid-Maine Medical Center, in Waterville. "O.K.?"

"I guess so."

Forrest West, in a green shirt and green hopsacking trousers with a broad leather belt, could be a forest ranger. He wears moccasins and no tie. He has tousled hair, a soothing mustache, dark eyes, and a speaking tone so calm and quiet it may occupy a frequency of its own. Paul Forman, tall and slim, is the more emotional and animated of the two. He comes to work wearing a short-sleeved shirt, a tie, a railroad engineer's cap, and, like West, puts on no white coat, no office paraphernalia to suggest his medical authority. On West's desk is an antique wooden box with gold scroll lettering that says, "West's Excelsior Veterinary Remedies." Forman could have stepped out of the cab of a train.

Forman and West have six thousand people in their catchment area. After five years, they include in their folders twenty-three hundred families. When they first approached the six towns, it was with some worry, although the situation in many ways appeared to fit their ideals. They listened to the people closely, trying to discern the extent to which they might be believers in the myth of the old Superdoc and be hoping for his return. With modern roads and modern populations, even in rural Maine a doctor could be overworked to the point of burning out. Forman and West found, to their relief, that the people of the towns were much aware of the difference, and were not expecting miracles—just a service the towns did not have.

Now Forman addresses a neighbor who has come in to discuss the results of a blood test. It shows an elevation in levels of serum glutamic-oxaloacetic transaminase, serum glutamic-pyruvic transaminase, lactic dehydrogenase. A question that has arisen in Forman's mind is not complicated by variable diagnosis. He says, "How much are you drinking?"

"Like I told you, I drink only ten beers a week."

"And how much hard stuff?"

"Don't touch it."

"How about carbon tetrachloride?"

"Don't touch it."

"Do you think you could give up alcohol?"

"I sure do. Wouldn't bother me a bit."

"Stay off alcohol for two months."

In Exam Room 3, Forrest West sets a Doppler microphone on the rising abdomen of Jane Glidden, whose second child is halfway along between conception and birth. She is twenty-three, works as a waitress, is married to a machinist, and lives in a house trailer in Palermo. Her mother, her father, her grandparents, and her year-old son are all patients of Dr. West's. A year ago, she came in to the clinic after two hours of labor, and—with time having run out for a trip to the hospital —her baby was born in Exam Room 3. The Doppler is turned on, and the new baby broadcasts loudly from the womb. It is the sound of a chorus of swamp frogs.

A mother brings in a child with a perforated eardrum. Forman asks her why she did not go to an otolaryngologist.

She says, "I figured you guys could do just as well as he could, and a lot cheaper."

The perforation is long-standing, not infected. For-man says, "I think you ought to see an ear specialist to follow that along."

Chris McMorrow next, thirty years old, a patient of Forman's who cannot eat lobster because afterward his throat always burns—an abysmal handicap in Maine. On this visit, McMorrow complains of a persis-tent headache and a crick in the neck. These symptoms may or may not be related to his eighteen-speed moun-tain bike, a leg-driven balloon-tired machine that is geared for roadless areas, including mountainsides. Last weekend, McMorrow went biking on Mt. Katahdin. Forman tells him that his trapezius muscle, in spasm, is producing the headaches by hauling on his scalp. The medical way to deal with the problem is with aspirin, or with stronger drugs—also by strengthening the muscle or by avoiding the use of it for purposes that tax it. Another approach is chiropractic—having to do with a possible pinched nerve in a vertebra—and Forman says that that helps some people. He says he is not as down on chiropractors as many doctors are, because he has friends that chiropractic has helped. Forman goes on to explain to McMorrow that osteopathy is a mixture of medical and manipulation techniques. Categorically, he will not cast aspersion on either profession. "Make an appointment if you wish."

Esten Peabody—white-bearded and fifty-one—comes in full of potato chips, which he professes to find irresistible. He is also full of good news: he has donated a pint of blood, and his blood pressure has dropped below the danger level.

Forman says, "We'll have to go back to using leeches." He also tells Peabody a thing or two about his diet, and reminds him of the silent progress of hypertension: "You don't feel bad until you have a stroke or your kidneys rot out. It's an asymptomatic disease."

Warren Harding, sixty-two, walks in slowly, sits down, and delivers to Forrest West a lecture on subverted justice—case after case dismissed because confessions were felt to be coerced. West listens. "We are throwing out the United States Constitution to protect criminals," Warren Harding tells him, and then asks, without a pause, "Will I get better? Will I ever get any strength back in my left arm?" Harding is an Albion farmer. For reasons unexplained, there is a closed safety pin hanging in the middle of his T-shirt.

West says to him, "When a stroke stabilizes for this length of time, things don't change."

West grew up in suburban Philadelphia, Forman in Pittsfield, Massachusetts. They went to small, northerly colleges (Williams and Hamilton) and to first-rate medical schools (Jefferson and Albany) on their way to Maine. When Forman was still in medical school, he wrote down his goals as a physician, and although he did not know Forrest West, he could have been speaking for him, too. He said he wanted "to develop a well-rounded understanding of medicine" so that he could "approach the patient as a whole person" whose physical problems often arise from emotional and social causes. He wished "to teach people about their own health, allay their fears about mild problems, counsel and guide them through seemingly complex treatment regimens when their problems are more serious"—all in a context of "compassionate, *high-quality* medicine." The italics were his. He wanted to seek a place where he was really needed, in order to "avoid being just another specialist competing for a limited number of cases," and he particularly hoped to find it "in an area with high mountains, cold white winters, and people who love and respect the natural resources available to them." He wrote that ten years ago, when he was twenty-five. Now he and his family live on a smoothly scraped dirt road and own twenty-three acres of high, forested land. From the deck of their house one can see long distances into some of the most beautiful country in Maine. Dari Forman, the doctor's wife, is a carpenter and custom furnituremaker, and she designed and built the house—a rhythmic geometry of heavy beams and bright glass composed with regard to the sun. Hemlock rafters, pine siding, elm-and-cherry stairway—she chose the rough lumber and had it milled. With dry pegs she joined green beams, which developed beauty as they checked. Insufficiently impressed by her wood stove and her passive-solar installations, the mortgagee bank—being a Maine bank, and not a Las Vegas drive-in—insisted on alternative electric-baseboard heat. Even with outside air at twenty below, the electric heat has never been needed.

Her husband repairs canoes, flies sailplanes, makes

house calls. "Some families are suspicious of doctors," he says. "And especially of young whippersnappers. A house call can help persuade them to come in." As Forman and West drive through the countryside from one to another of the six towns, they connect patients' faces to a high percentage of the names on the mailboxes. They believe in "one-on-one doctor-patient relationships," and they believe in availability (to the maximum extent that the concerns of "the doctor's family and the doctor's mental health" will permit). Always, they leave open two morning and two afternoon appointments, so that no patient in difficulty will call their number and be given the classic American sentence "The next open appointment is in December." After five years, Forman and West are functioning near the extreme margins of these criteria, and they would be pleased to be joined by a third physician. It would have to be someone, though, who shares their "definition of emergency," which they give in the form of an example: a patient who calls up at midnight with sore throat. "Unless such patients are chronic abusers, you go and see them. They have been miserable enough to make the call."

Toward noon one day, West gets into his car to drive twelve miles to the hospital in Waterville and make a house call en route. He listens to cassettes as he makes these journeys, listens hundreds of hours per year. The cassette of the moment is called "Dermatology Update —Scabies, Anogenital Skin Disease, and Psoriasis." Forman listens to similar tapes in his car. To keep up with things, they also rely on conversations with specialists they know and trust. They read three or four medical journals and throw the rest out. Perhaps to a higher degree than on any other type of doctor, pressure is on the family practitioner to keep up with developing medical knowledge, for fear that one's capability quotient will drop below the multivalent stratum and into the dilettante zone. Various specialists and subspecialists who do not look upon family practitioners as people with a Renaissance range of application and knowledge will undercut them more on the matter of keeping up than on any other, saying, typically, that medical knowledge "explodes every five years" or "increases five per cent a year and therefore doubles every fourteen years," and that almost no one in any subspecialty can ingest enough of the new information, let alone a generalist whose pretense to competence spans many fields.

Disagreement being an apparent norm in medical dialogue, it is not difficult to find specialists who beg to differ:

"It *is* possible to know a broad swath of medicine."

"It's simply not true that medicine explodes every five years. You can generally get along on old practices."

"In terms of day-to-day care of people, quite frankly, you don't have to keep up. Diseases haven't changed that much. People's emotions haven't changed that much. Except for status, family practitioners don't have to keep up with a good many things. Technology is the kudzu of medicine. It's choking all of us. There are so many technological things we don't need. If you look at hospital mortality rates—the number of patients who come in, the number who die, the number who go home—they have not really changed in thirty years."

Another way to keep up—and get a free meal at the same time—is to attend, say, a peritonitis conference in a hospital lunchroom. The atmosphere in such places tends to be smoky, collegial, and varied, involving large percentages of the staff. Tomorrow is phlebitis. Meanwhile, the peritonitis charts are barely legible through the smoke. That big gentleman in the green tunic and green cap—the man with the hacking cough, the chain Marlboros, and the Hawaiian paunch—is a thoracic surgeon.

West turns into the driveway of the old farmhouse of Franklin Whitman. West drapes his stethoscope around his neck, picks up his black leather medical bag, and goes into the house through the kitchen entrance. He greets Everett Whitman, who is about fifty, and Everett's mother, Florence, and walks through the kitchen into a parlor that is crowded with the accumulations of uncounted years. Deeply piled on tables and cabinets are stacks of magazines tied with string. There are many cardboard cartons, some open, and miscellaneously filled. Where the wallpaper is lesioned, plaster is loose upon the lath of the walls—over a sewing machine that was new before the first Ford. Stuffed chairs are slipcovered with blankets. On a central table, a cat rests at the apex of a pyramid of boxes and magazines. As West enters, the cat leaps away, knocking over a glass, and the beverage inside flows and drips off the magazines and table to the floor. The room is generously heated. Franklin Whitman, seventy-four years old, lies on a couch with blankets drawn over his chin. A bald head and horn-rimmed glasses are about all that can be seen of him, and an obvious shiver. He is pleased to see West, and says so, despite his acute discomfort—his classic erratic chills and fever, picket-fence in pattern, which overlie chronic suffering from acute arthritis. As West listens to his heart, and listens to and notes his blood pressure, Whitman's wife and son stand in the doorway and watch. The blood pressure goes down when the patient sits up. Flu? Septicemia? West has been here several times in recent days. Whitman is on steroids, and they suppress the immune reaction. Has a bacterial infection developed in his blood? West decides to admit him, and explains to all three why the hospital at this point seems the place for the patient to be. As he leaves, Florence Whitman, who is elderly and fragile, too, says to him in a vibrant voice, "Thank you for coming, Doctor. Thank you for coming so soon."

West drives to Waterville—to the Mid-Maine Medical Center, and, within the complex, to a hospital of largely fresh construction, its sparkling corridors and heavy silent doors imparting a sense of order and, with it, an implication that this place is still on the innocent side of the creeping chaos that seems to advance with time on even the most impressively pedigreed of medical institutions. At a nurses' station, West looks over some charts, some radiological reports, preparing to see his patients. The first is Seth Fuller, whose X-rays now reveal the collapse of a small segment of lung—left and low. Possible causes include but are not limited to a swollen lymph node, a tumor, the aspiration of something or other. "Remember," he comments, "there is always a chance that it is something benign, with a good prognosis."

West goes to Fuller's bedside. Fuller is sitting up, eyes missing nothing, talking quietly with his wife, his daughter, and her husband. Now and again, he coughs —a low dry cough. The *Central Maine Morning Sentinel* is on the bed by his elbow: "WALESA WINS NOBEL PRIZE," "WHITE SOX, DODGERS WIN PLAYOFF GAMES." A bearded, barrel-chested man lies anonymously in the next bed, looking away from the Fuller tableau and out a wide window into a sunlighted October day, rock maples in blaze—a day as bright and crisp and indigenous as West's patient in bed. Fuller is active in the Grange. One year, when the state was offering fruit trees in Winslow, Fuller went over and picked up a load of trees for West. West tells him about the X-rays and reviews the list of possibilities, his slow voice flat and calm. The two say nothing for a while—in a communicative and unawkward silence, each relying (with a confidence long since developed) on the other. Eventually, West says, "Sometimes, if you have a tumor and it's localized in a small area you can treat it by taking it out."

Fuller says nothing for a time, and then says, "Some fellows get along with just one lung. I had a neighbor had just one lung. He was awful short of breath. He couldn't walk uphill for nothin'."

Again, time passes gracefully while neither West nor Fuller speaks. Finally, West says, "O.K.?"

And Fuller says, "O.K. I'll be right here, then."

Sixteen-year-old female comes in for a blood count. This is not Albion. This is anywhere, any day and every day, in the pan-Maine family-practice clinical montage. She is petite and lovely, with silky brown hair. Her fingernails are long, and the paint is chrome. She is a junior in high school, and has come straight from class to the doctor's office, wearing a bright-blue maternity gown with the word "BABY" in large block letters under the throat. The baby is due in about a week. If it is male, the doctor asks, is he to be circumcised?

"What is that?" asks the patient.

After explaining circumcision, the doctor has another question. Is the baby to be born in the hospital's birthing room or the delivery room (the birthing room being, more or less, a simulated home bedroom)?

"I haven't heard bad things about neither one of them," the patient says, with a shrug.

The doctor places a stethoscope on the stretched-to-shining skin above the womb. The baby sounds like a carpenter pounding on a roof.

The doctor remarks, after the patient has gone, "More often than not, around here, kids carry their babies and keep them. We see kids like that quite often. No birth control. She's never used it."

Nineteen-year-old female, shy in manner and proud of her children, brings them in together for pediatric checkups. One is two months old, the other two years old. They have different fathers. Their mother has never been married.

Seventeen-year-old female, unmarried, comes in with her toddler son, who has an ear infection. She conceived and bore him in another part of the country and came to Maine with the baby to live with her sister and complete her high-school education. The sister, who is twenty-one years old and unmarried, is pregnant.

"I went to Portland twice a week for a month to learn to do abortions," the doctor remarks after one teenager and her child have gone. "I almost couldn't take it. All those young women. Some of their reasons for doing it disgusted me. I even called in sick one day. I happen to think that putting a baby up for adoption is a better choice to make, but I believe that abortion is an option that should be offered. Some people actually carry babies in order to have the state support them and their boyfriends. They live off their babies." The State of Maine pays about two hundred and seventy dollars a month to a single mother with one child, and for each additional child increases the support.

A grandmother, a mother, and a two-week-old baby come in. All three are patients of this doctor, as is the baby's grandfather. The new mother wears a blue shirt, running shoes, jeans. She is sixteen and a sophomore in high school. She has told the name of the father to no one.

"Have you been feeling blue or down in the dumps?" the doctor asks her.

Almost inaudibly, she says, "No."

The doctor says to her, "Sometimes people do after they've had a baby."

"I'll be going back to school on Tuesday."

"Who takes care of the baby then?"

"I do," says the young mother's mother. "It's been a long time since I've had a little baby in the house."

Next, a thirty-eight-year-old female in her third pregnancy.

Doctor: "Is everything O.K.?"

Patient: "You're the doctor. You tell me."

"Do you drink milk?"

"I like milk if it has Kahlua in it."

"What else do you drink?"

"Sometimes a couple of beers."

"Smoke?"

"Pack a day for twenty years."

"Caffeine?"

"None."

"Cats?"

"Three."

"How much do you happen to know about toxo-plasmosis in pregnancy?"

Fifty-nine-year-old female, in slacks and running shoes, says she has come in to discuss her arthritis. Her gnarled fingers sparkle with gemstones. After a time, the doctor says, "So for now you want to stick with aspirin?" He knows, though, that she is not here to talk about aspirin, or even her chronic headaches, for which she takes Elavil. She is here just to talk, as she has been in the past and will be in the future, and he is more than prepared to listen. Two relatives of her husband live in her home; each is retarded and needs quite special care. As time has passed, the situation has grown in various ways less tolerable to her. There is nothing the doctor can prescribe except his time, his interest, and his watchful sympathy—all of which she receives.

Fifteen-year-old female presents with a history of dizziness, fainting, difficulty sleeping, and apparent anorexia. She reports that she never eats lunch, never eats dinner, and has cereal in the morning under a blizzard of sugar. Her mother is with her and nods—it's a fact. The patient is sexually active. The doctor offers birth-control pills. The mother, with anguish in her face, agrees. That is all the doctor will offer, however. The patient has twice attempted suicide. The doctor recommends that someone more specifically trained should be listening to her.

Seventy-five-year-old female presents with a problem list that would impress a laundry. Heart disease, cataracts, emphysema, a sore rib . . . She smokes, by her count, twenty cigarettes a day. Twice, she has nearly died. A month ago, she came in with shortness of breath and incipient heart failure. The doctor sees her regularly, knows her well, and today can let the large matters go.

"How you doing?"

"Up and down. I can't walk far. My rib hurts, and my head has a burning itch."

"The people next door there, they have lice, you know."

"I know that. I don't go over there. I don't like the smell over there."

"You know them well?"

"He's my nephew."

"Does he help you?"

"He don't help nothing."

The doctor finds bites on her legs but not on her scalp. Her cough has the sound of a hatchet. She gets up to leave. "Can I see you in about a month?" the doctor says.

Patient says, "Make it in the forenoon, please."

A fifty-two-year-old female comes in and encapsulates her presenting complaint in four short words: "I just feel blah." As Sandy Burstein noted, the family practitioner generally has less to begin with than, say, a nephrologist, who knows when referrals come in that their problems are in their kidneys. "Blah" is a psychomedical condition at the center of square one, and that is where the family practitioner's diagnosis begins.

Sixteen-year-old male comes in for a school physical, mandatory for athletes in contact sports. He is sharply featured, handsome. Blondish hair tumbles toward his dark eyes. His ambition is to join the United States Marine Corps, and meanwhile he runs long distances, lifts weights, plays football, and has reached advanced levels in acrobatic karate. He has smoked since age eleven, and he has one breast that has developed fully in female form. Listening to his heart, the doctor tells him that he has a slight, unimportant murmur, and offhandedly says about the breast, "It doesn't mean you are not a man. It's a thing that happens to teen-agers. It means you are becoming a man. Do you notice, in sports, that your smoking affects you—that you have less strength?"

"Nope. It never has—as long as I keep in good shape and keep on running."

"If you ever have a heart attack, you'll have less chance of surviving. Do you use drugs?"

"You don't have to talk to me about that. I don't touch 'em."

"Alcohol?"

"No."

"If you continue smoking, you won't feel different until maybe sixty per cent of your lungs are gone."

"Well, I could quit."

Fifty-two-year-old male—a new patient—has recently suffered a subarachnoid hemorrhage and now seeks post-operative care. He also seeks counsel. His twenty-five-year-old unmarried daughter, who works at Dunkin' Donuts, has no apparent intention of leaving home and meanwhile is steadily gaining weight—expanding like nut dough—and has become, in her father's words, "a pain in the ass." In response to suggestions or criticism, her usual reply is "It's my life."

"Yes," the doctor says. "But it's your house."

Across the patient's face comes a look of gratitude. "People up here worry a lot about not having doctors," he says. "I'm so glad you're willing to take on my case."

Telephone rings. There is a patient up the road whom the doctor sees only on house calls, for she has long been in a coma and has not opened her eyes in five years. Living with her and caring for her are her son and two other men. They have bought a hospital bed and placed it in the center of the parlor, which they routinely adorn with fresh flowers. They keep the room airy, dustless, and clean. They feed the patient with an eyedropper. Month in, year out, they give her loving, intensive care. Now her son is on the phone with a question for the doctor. Would it be all right if he and the others took his mother on a camping trip?

Old Superdoc might have got along on the contents of his black bag, but a modern country doctor, in order to function effectively, needs a close relationship with a hospital. The hospital does not have to be Massachusetts General. It can be modest in all its dimensions and nonetheless be prepared to handle ninety-eight per cent of the cases that arise within its catchment area. A good community hospital somewhere nearby is all a family practitioner needs, other than an office and a neatly lettered sign. As it happens, though, not all community hospitals feel an equal need for the family practitioner.

A doctor setting up a practice does not simply call up the nearest hospital and start admitting patients. The doctor must formally obtain privileges to do so, and from field to field the privileges are discrete—obstetrical privileges, surgical privileges, medical privileges. Privileges are controlled by the hospital staff, which consists of doctors. In England, doctors who work in hospitals are not the same doctors who work in the community, and patients are transferred from the one milieu to the other. In the United States, of course, the doctors who are out in offices getting the first look at the business are, by and large, also on the hospital staff. If a new doctor comes into a town and the new doctor's type of training augurs competition for one or more people on the hospital's staff, the established doctors can, in effect, tie off the newcomer's tubes. The procedure is more formally described as denying privileges. The situation can be difficult for any new specialist, but when a doctor comes along who has been board-certified to function up to various levels of obstetrics, gynecology, pediatrics, internal medicine, dermatology, otolaryngology, and a dozen or two related subspecialties, someone on the staff is almost surely going to mutter about "the need to preserve high standards," and someone else, inevitably, will slide his glasses down his nose, peer out over the rims, and say, "Let's look at those credentials a little more closely." This is known in medical anthropology as the battle for turf. It is one aspect of medicine that most patients can follow at least as comprehendingly as their doctors, because the battle for turf is where doctors display their commonality with the rest of humankind, where they mirror most closely the society they serve, where the snakes come off the caduceus and the one makes a meal of the other.

Turf.

"Do you need a cardiologist or a gastroenterologist for a heart attack or an ulcer?" asks a family practitioner. "That is the question, and in most cases the answer is no. We're on their turf, and for the most part we can handle their problems as well as they can. They try to restrict what we can do. At the same time, they try to be nice to us so they can get our referrals."

Turf extends to such matters as the reading of electrocardiograms, on which a local cardiologist will often have a monopoly, and for which third-party payers —insurance companies, governments—pay well. So the hospital, in a manner of speaking, has decided that while it is permissible for family practitioners to look at their own patients' EKGs, the EKGs must be "overread" by the cardiologist "in order to preserve the hospital's high standards." Moreover, family practitioners are often denied privileges to look after their own patients in coronary-care units. In many hospitals, it is equally difficult for family practitioners to obtain privileges in obstetrics, or to function in intensive care. In the words of one grizzled internist, "So these kids get frozen out of everything they've been taught to do and they wind up having no real privileges at all. This happens a good deal in sophisticated little towns." In large cities, turf battles are often so intense they are virtually audible, and family practitioners can be given so few privileges that even patients come to regard them as glorified nurses. As a result, some family practitioners shrug their shoulders and go into storefront medicine, a modern phenomenon whereby doctors do business in former shoe stores and pet shops, treating customers who walk in off the street. There are chains, with franchises—agglomerately nick-named Doc in a Box—where you can use your Master-Card to cover your treatment for hypoglycemia or bubonic plague.

Turf battles of another kind, and of epic proportions, frequently occur between hospitals, whose rivalries can be even more intense than the rivalries among the doctors who work in them. Even the spread-out hospitals of a state like Maine float in their drainage catchments like ships of war, and fire salvos at one another beyond the horizons. They compete fiercely for customers. Jealously, they guard their relationships with peripheral towns. Ironically, the more intense such regional warfare becomes, the more it favors the family practitioners. Hospitals even support them out there, the better to defend their sphere.

Not all turf battles end unhappily. When Ann Dorney was completing her residency, she and several colleagues studied a map of their Maine surroundings, gathered parameters of various kinds—size and quality of hospitals, relative need for doctors, proximity to the coastal fjords, proximity to the Great North Woods—

and tugged and pulled and debated one another until they descended *en groupe* upon Skowhegan. With one exception, these doctors were women—they would ultimately include four women—and they wanted to practice together.

Skowhegan, on the Kennebec River, is a town of eight thousand people forty miles upstream from Augusta, twenty from Waterville. Among the people are pulpers, debarkers, last-pullers. It is a timbering and shoe-factory red brick town, where fights break out on Saturday nights and serenity usually characterizes the rest of the week. Madison Paper Industries is close to Skowhegan, and *The New York Times Magazine* is literally standing there, too, with little cones hanging from its branches—not to mention the needles. With Athens and Canaan, Madison and Norridgewock, the catchment of Skowhegan's Redington-Fairview General Hospital is twenty-four thousand people, and the setting of farmland and forest, moose country, bear country, appealed to these particular doctors no less than the promising medical factors. The hospital was well equipped and had ninety-two beds. There were four internists, a pediatrician, five surgeons, and two general practitioners nearing retirement. An obstetrician had recently died, and another had left town. There had been a turf battle over whether to seek specialists or family practitioners to join the medical staff. When Dorney and the others made their interest known, various doctors on the hospital staff were at first opposed, fearing the competitive numbers. A turf skirmish followed, lacking the intensity of a full-scale battle but crucial nonetheless, and culminating in a dramatic encounter between the young family practitioners and the established physicians of Skowhegan. Initially, it appeared that Skowhegan was going to ask the family practitioners to establish themselves in peripheral towns, but in the evolving discussion the older doctors changed their minds. One of them went outside and yanked up a piece of the hospital lawn. Returning to the meeting, he gave the hunk of sod to the young doctors, and said, "O.K., here is a piece of our turf."

Next door to the hospital, at 34 Fairview Avenue, was an old rambling house—a wide porch, wood siding, two stories, a steep gable roof—and the hospital bought it for the use of the new doctors. Two or three of their husbands happened to be, among other things, carpenters, and they turned the front parlor into a waiting room, the dining room into a reception room, the kitchen into a lab. Ann Dorney—who had been raised in Green Bay, Wisconsin, by a mother who taught home economics—sewed gowns and drape sheets for patients, made curtains for the exam-room windows, and covered cushions and made eight-foot draperies for the waiting room. By seeking out retired physicians all over central Maine, the group found antique examining tables of teak and mahogany, and corner cabinetry of similar construction. The house, under big rock maples, stands in the center of a lovely, breezy scene—set back among lawns near the edge of open country. A wooden placard by the patients' entrance says:

SKOWHEGAN FAMILY MEDICINE
DAVID AXELMAN, M.D.
ANN DORNEY, M.D.
DONNA CONKLING, M.D.
SUSAN COCHRAN, M.D.
CYNTHIA ROBERTSON, M.D.

In their residency days, these people were known
—for their sensitivity to global ecology, their affection
for wild country, their medically defensive gourmandise
—as the Granola Group. Now in medical circles in
Skowhegan they are sometimes called David's Girls.
Outside the old house are some aging automobiles of
which it could be said that there would be nothing
ethically amiss if they were permitted to roll over and
put their wheels in the air. These are the physicians'
cars. They closely resemble the groaning heaps in which
many of their patients come to see them. Like most of
their former Maine–Dartmouth colleagues, the young
doctors of Skowhegan tend to dress no more formally
than the people they examine. They wear bluejeans,
bluejean skirts. David Axelman is likely to be wearing
a cotton cambric shirt, corduroy jeans, and ankle-high
boots as he examines a patient in a cotton cambric shirt,
corduroy jeans, and ankle-high boots. Axelman, who is
Jewish, refuses to do circumcisions. As a boy in Philadelphia, he developed a phobia about circumcisions, and
did not expunge the phobia at the Medical College of
Pennsylvania. Ann Dorney does his circumcisions for
him. She also does most vasectomies for the group.

Dr. Dorney is a slender woman whose auburn hair is allowed to stream down her back but only after paying toll at a barrette. In manner, she seems diffident, but she expresses without hesitation just what she thinks and feels. Colleagues and teachers have long singled her out for her speed of decision, her mastery of techniques, and her quiet confidence. She was born in Ladysmith, Wisconsin. She is a Phi Beta Kappa from Earlham College, in Richmond, Indiana. Thirty now, she was twenty-four and still in the medical school of George Washington University when she wrote in an application, "I am extremely responsible." With an autobiography like that, and a predilection for rimless spectacles, she could be cast as a cameo schoolmarm, but in fact she lacks severity and could not fill the role. Her smile is warm and as informal as her autumn-colored blouses, sleeveless cardigans, corduroy skirts, and leather sandals. She is a cyclist, a backpacker, a canoe-tripper, and she is actively concerned about nuclear energy, nuclear weaponry, and lesser environmental issues. She knits, sews, cans vegetables, does occasional carpentry, and sees in the office about sixty patients a week, others each morning on hospital rounds. In all the range of patients, she likes most to see older males, because they present with heart disease, diabetes, troubles in the prostate gland— conditions that interest her especially. Female patients, however, come in large numbers to her—to her and to Donna Conkling and to Sue Cochran and to Cynthia Robertson, because they are women. Over the lakes and out of the forests, off every kind of farm—jumping over catchment areas, ignoring larger hospitals, bypassing established medical tycoons—women seek the women of Skowhegan. Women come from Waterville. They come from beyond Augusta. They bring children and husbands with them. The Skowhegan group in its first ten months of practice wrote folders for a thousand families. "Some days it's all G.Y.N., or all peds and G.Y.N.," Dorney has complained. "My goal in medicine is a truly general practice."

The size of their practice notwithstanding, as businesswomen (and businessman) these Skowhegan doctors can fairly be placed on Flake 9. They have had as much as fifty thousand dollars in accounts receivable and scarcely enough cash to buy their own food. At the end of the day at 34 Fairview Avenue, the doctors empty the wastebaskets and sweep the floor. Once a week, after hours, they have a group meeting. Sue Cochran—elongate, high-strung, swift of humor—sprawls on a couch in the reception room and breast-feeds her son, Matthiah. Cynthia Robertson, as trig as a flight attendant, is down from Bingham—twenty-four miles into the woods— where she works three days a week, discharging an obligation to the Public Health Service that she incurred to pay for her medical education. Donna Conkling— easygoing, unhurried, serene in manner—comes in and sets down her shoulder bag. It is made from a pair of overalls. The straps go over her shoulder. The legs have been amputated and sutured at the thighs. After sitting down, she nurses her son Will. Axelman does not assert himself with these women. He is a long, loosely as-

sembled, bearded, and colloquial man with wide interested eyes suggesting a mind that requires no mask. It
was decided at one of these meetings that obstetrical patients must be limited to twelve a month or the group
might soon have a practice that was nothing much but
O.B.–G.Y.N. At another meeting, after less than a year
in practice, they discussed limiting the total number of
patients of any kind, so large had the practice become.
At these meetings, the conversation is not in Latin.
Terms such as "weirdo" and "berserko"—and "like" as
like an adverb—vastly outnumber such terms as "reticu-
lation," "auscultation," and "contraindicated."

After serious matters have been dealt with, the
really serious matters arise for discussion:

"Who took my wastebasket?"

"My tape measure has disappeared from my exam-
ination room."

"I can't find my alcohol bottle."

Once a month, the meeting is expanded to include
the doctors' significant others. This is known as an S.O.
meeting. Dorney is divorced and Axelman has never
married, but the others' significant others include Sue
Cochran's husband, David Larkin, who is a carpenter
in Skowhegan and is studying theology in Bangor; Bob
Conkling, who is also a part-time carpenter; and Cynthia
Robertson's husband, Bob McLaughlin. The two Bobs
are scholars of varied dimension, experts on Maine Indians (Conkling has a degree in anthropology), and
together they spent six months in training at the Augusta Mental Health Institute and additional time with

a counsellor in Bangor in order to prepare to talk with patients whose physical complaints might be reduced through psychological counsel. In an upstairs room in the old house, they offer dual therapy.

"The practice is too big—we're having to run them through like cattle," Sue Cochran remarks. Of all people, she is not exactly in a position to complain. She once stopped a family in a supermarket and recruited them as patients. She was drawn to them because they included two adopted children—one from Colombia, the other from El Salvador. When she was an undergraduate at Radcliffe, she took a course taught by Harvard medical students on the subject of corruption in American medicine. It eroded some of her familial, knee-spasm respect for the profession, and also started her on the way to her eventual conclusion that an American medical education is incomplete. She describes herself now as "cool toward the curative approach." She will explain, "Not enough is studied about how the body keeps well. Medicine treats symptoms and doesn't get at causes. Studying disease is a backward way to do medicine. When you treat an ulcer, you're not treating what caused it. Teaching such things to a patient should be ninety per cent of the practice of medicine. It's not—as done by most people. In the education of a doctor, finishing an orthodox residency ought to be only the first step. We have training, but not enough. I would like to learn acupuncture. We should be making full evaluations of all patients—their life styles, habits, dietary preferences. Asians do it. We should be doing it, too."

Donna Conkling, a birthright Quaker who grew up near Philadelphia, taught English in Celebes while her husband did research there. She contracted amoebic dysentery and was so sick that she experienced each of the classic stages of dying (shock and denial, anger, bargaining, depression, preparatory grief . . .) except the last. After returning to the United States, she prepared for and entered the Medical College of Pennsylvania. During her final year, she went to Maine to be interviewed by the Augusta residency and was impressed by the faculty's welcoming reaction to the fact that she was pregnant. Spontaneously, the director outlined for her various ways in which a second child could be planned during her time in the residency. "Just as I had used family practice as a divining rod for choosing a medical school, I used my big belly as a divining rod for a residency," she would say later. Augusta became her first choice, and meanwhile she rode her bicycle through the streets of Philadelphia almost up to the moment of the birth of Joel Conkling, then took six weeks off to get him started, returned to the medical college, and finished with her class. It helped that Bob Conkling had gone out of anthropology and into carpentry, working on urban construction jobs. He stayed home to look after Joel. In Maine, he and David Larkin built an envelope house on land in Vassalboro that belonged to Ann Dorney. Everybody moved in. They grew their own vegetables under glass through the coldest weather. The envelope was so well sealed that they heated the place through the winter on less than half a cord of wood.

The Conklings, four in all, now live in a cabin up a trail in forest twelve miles from Skowhegan—a setting not unlike the bush-country homesteads of Alaska. Axelman and Dorney are out in the moose range, too, as are Sue Cochran, David Larkin, and Matthiah, who have been living beside a fire pit and a running brook, in a wall tent made of polyethylene sheets, on eighty acres of stunning land, where Larkin is constructing a house. Sue Cochran daydreams that someday all the doctors might live together again, on this property, and have "little pathways between houses, and stuff." In the office and hospital, meanwhile, she and Donna Conkling are attempting to work things out so that they share the equivalent of one full practice and retain the balance of their time to raise their children. The experiment is being watched with interest by physicians elsewhere in Maine, who, variously, believe that the idea is a good one or think it impossible to be a part-time doctor.

The pace of the practice as it has developed in Skowhegan is especially alarming to Donna Conkling. To see twenty or twenty-five patients in a day is not her idea of family practice. "I don't see myself as ever seeing that many patients," she says. "I'm too interested in learning what people's lives are like."

Ann Dorney does not have a lot of choice about how many people she sees in a day. She is there all the time, and patients keep coming through the door. Before they begin appearing, she makes rounds in Redington-Fairview—sees Deborah Kratzsch, for example, whose baby, Alan, is a few days old. Dorney touches Alan's cheek. His mouth forms an O and turns toward her hand. He is ready to suck. "That's the rooting reflex," Dorney comments. "Older people with strokes can have the rooting reflex, too."

Nellie Burns has a fast-growing tumor in her stomach which is beyond the skill of surgery. The two women, one of them aged thirty, the other seventy-five, begin a remarkably relaxed conversation—Dorney straightforward, her patient receptive and not alarmed.

"You have to think about what you are going to do. For instance, you have to think about where you want to die."

"How much time might there be?"

"It could be within a month."

"I will die at home."

In the corridor, Dorney remarks that cancer was diagnosed in both Nellie Burns and her husband at about the same time. Dorney stops at the bedside of Elizabeth Easler, seventy-seven, who came into the hospital with a myocardial infarction and suffered another heart attack—actually, an extension of the first one—four days later. Rounds completed, Dorney remarks that Redington-Fairview has equipment that some people might not expect—all sorts of things, from temporary pacemakers to Swan-Ganz catheters. "The quality of care can be every bit as good in a place like this as in a big-city hospital. The risk of a small hospital is that a poor physician can have more effect. A good one, on the other hand, can do more, and therefore be more effective. In a small hospital, quality of care can be easily changed by the coming or going of a couple of people. If you have good people, you can do wonders."

After walking from the hospital to the old clapboard house under the rock maples, she is involved right away with a two-week-old baby who has an infected navel, then a debarker's wife whose baby is due in four weeks, then a twenty-four-year-old man who presents with general fatigue. He is a last-puller in one of the shoe shops—as shoe factories are known in Maine. For two years, this gentleman's complete job description has been "pulling one shoe after another off a last." After he leaves, Dorney remarks, "Who would not complain of being tired?"

Ten-year-old male with allergy problems. When his father first brought him in, Dorney asked at length about the family's history, and the father happened to remark that now and again he took his own blood pressure. The last time he did so, he got a hundred and seventy over a hundred and ten. "Wow!" she said, and wrapped his arm and squeezed the bulb. A hundred and seventy over a hundred and ten. Subsequently, she discovered that he had adult-onset diabetes and was developing angina. Without the prescriptions and treatment that followed, the man would in all likelihood have died —as his brother had recently—of a myocardial infarction. It was a sequence of familial treatment that might not have happened in another kind of office.

85

A forty-four-year-old female, her weight in excess of three hundred pounds, presents herself to Dr. Dorney. The two are together for the better part of an hour. There are some prescriptions, a gift of sample cream. After the patient leaves, Dorney says, "That was the first complete physical and pelvic exam she has ever had."

A twelve-year-old male presents with a large hydrocele around one testicle. To be sure that that is what it is, Dorney transilluminates it. His mother, standing by, says she would like to know, just out of curiosity, if a baby can be made with one testicle. The answer is affirmative. The mother has a second question: "Can a man make a baby if he's been smoking pot?"

Asked how often she sees something in her practice that she did not see in her training, Dorney says, "About once a month. Most recently, it was umbilical cellulitis. We picked up all kinds of unusual things when we first came into the area. Most of our patients have not been transferring from other doctors."

One who did transfer was a twenty-six-year-old female with a right-side kidney stone, who came to Dorney after deciding that a urologist was no help. The patient appears now—jeans, running shoes, terry-cloth shirt. She has developed an infection. Given the presence of the stone, the infection makes Dorney uneasy, and she insists on involving a new urologist. "The stone itself can carry an infection," she explains after the patient leaves. "If it does, the stone must be removed. When a stone enters the ureter, there is severe pain. People writhe in pain, it's so bad. It's one of the worst pains there are."

Mary Doherty and Joe Niemczura come in—she a redhead, he with a full blond beard—five days before the due date of their first child. She is a nurse, and so is he. He is chief nurse in the Redington-Fairview intensive-care unit. His wife has developed preeclampsia— protein in her urine, high blood pressure, swelling. Her feet and hands are grossly swollen. All this can lead not only to problems with the placenta but also to seizures that could be fatal to the mother. "The idea now is to move fast, induce labor, and avoid the problems," says Dorney, and she writes on a hospital form, "39½ weeks gestation and preeclampsia, admitted for induction."

"But I'm not ready!" screams Joe Niemczura.

Mary Doherty contemplates Joe for a moment, and then, with an affectionate smile, says, "Go take the cats to the vet."

Still another gestating mother appears. She is near term. The stethoscope moves from place to place on the beehive womb. Variously, the child sounds like a locomotive, like a swimmer doing laps, like water gurgling in a drain. Dorney lays a cloth tape measure over the womb, pressing one end on the pubic bone. The number of centimetres from the pubic bone to the far side of the uterus equals the number of weeks of pregnancy, she says. "It's so consistent it's uncanny. If it's much farther, or short, the dates are probably off."

Even God is on the metric system.

JOHN McPHEE

When specialists talk about family practitioners and the family-practice movement, they tend not to speak as one.

"In the large teaching hospitals, we are essentially interlopers in people's lives. We rescue people from death's door and never see them again. Family practice is a very different form of medicine from what we practice."

"It dates from the mid-sixties, when the government began fiddling around too much with medicine. Now they are cutting down on the funding, and family practice may blow away. Let's hope so."

"Family practice is the most inspired medical movement to develop over the past fifteen years."

"It is a sad comment on the medical profession that it has not met the need without creating this polarization."

"The movement is political in origin and not medically based. It has been a social necessity and a professional disaster."

An obstetrician is likely to be quite negative, but not necessarily so, and a surgeon the reverse. They speak on various levels—the two principal strata being the level of medicine as science and the level of medicine as business. The one can be used to mask the other. An internist expressing antipathy to family practice may

88

simply be reacting to economic threat. An obstetrician mentioning points of science and technique may be masking fear of competition or, on the other hand, may be genuinely worried about family practitioners' dealing with obstetrical problems that are beyond the scope of their training. A surgeon speaking with enthusiasm about the family-practice movement and its 'benefits to society may be speaking essentially about its benefits to him. A family practitioner is a surgeon's travelling sales-man. In its fifteen years of formal existence, the family-practice "specialty" has been enduringly controversial in a profession where controversy seems to be the custom of the day and the interacting specialties are roughly as disputatious as lawyers are litigious.

The assembled dialogue that follows consists of comments, remarks, and explanatory anecdotes spoken or written by one or two medical students and physicians of various specialties and ages: doctors in Maine and in scattered other milieus, rural and suburban and city doctors—none of them in family practice.

"Say a patient has a heart attack and has two problems after he gets over it: he develops a dysrhythmia (he may be throwing ectopic beats) and he has a pain problem (he has angina from time to time). So he's on four different medications, some of which can interact in deleterious fashion. I don't think it's possible for the family practitioner to get that patient on all the proper drugs, because to do so takes an enormous amount of experience. You can't just read a book and then for A you give A prime and for B you give B prime. But once the patient is stabilized and is on those four medicines the cardiologist can send him back to his family practitioner and say, 'Here's the situation. You ought to see how he does, and maybe you want to increase his Inderal or drop his Norpace.' That is an appropriate way to deal with it. The family practitioner has to know about these four drugs—what their complications are, which ones will interact, which cardiac drug will synergize the effect of an anticoagulant and create a problem, which ones produce mental depression, which ones cause urinary retention. If you're on a bunch of medications and can't pee, you may not need a urologist, you may need to stop a drug. The family practitioner can do that. The family practitioner has to know things, but not in the same depth as subspecialists. It's the difference between a guy who's good at building an outhouse and a guy who can make a Queen Anne chair."

"It is sad that family practitioners have such a thin coating of high tech, which makes them marketable in a very limited field."

"They're like the Edsel. In its design, it was a good car, but its market was overestimated."

"Family medicine is a fad."

"Other physicians don't know what the role of the family practitioner is. Other physicians tend to think, Family practitioners can't know everything; therefore, they know nothing. The role of the family practitioner is *not* to know everything but to be a primary-care physician to a family, to provide continuity of health care from cradle to grave—a unique role in our society."

"People's expectations of what family practitioners will do are not real. For example, people want family doctors to come out and see them, but house calls are pointless. Family doctors are as high-tech as anyone else, and are probably making no more house calls than internists do. Maybe the family doctors can train their patients not to demand it. But the people who yearn for the good old family physician are the same people you hear saying, 'Damn, you just can't hire good help to clean up your house anymore.' "

"If you're a family practitioner, most of your people—over time, you know them. If Mrs. Smith calls and says she's having a heart attack, you may know from past experience that it's her angina and that she's probably had a fight with her husband. So you don't have to admit her to the hospital, put her in the coronary-care unit, and run up a big bill. Whereas if Mrs. Smith comes into the emergency department, where they've never seen her before, she doesn't say she has angina and had a fight with her husband, and it's three thousand bucks before you know it."

"Family practitioners do not have anything special to offer patients beyond a mix of superficially developed clinical skills."

"They do not possess much of the implicit information about patients and their families to which they lay claim in their self-descriptions."

"A woman takes her husband to an internist because he's been having chest pain—and after the checkup and the electrocardiogram the wife says, 'Oh, by the way, I have been having a vague belly pain.' That means the doctor is going to have to talk with her a little bit, and I think if it were anyone other than a family practitioner the matter would get sloughed off. 'Six weeks from Tuesday we have an open appointment'—you know what I mean. The family practitioner, though, is going to upset his schedule and settle that question right now, because he feels his commitment to take care of a family. All his appointments get pushed back, but he has a tendency to deal with such things then and there. It takes you a while to learn that following people in a longitudinal sense is the way to deal with both acute and chronic illness. None of us learn that as residents. Following people over time—rather than ordering a vast number of studies—is really the answer. Even as a surgeon, I find myself spending more time talking to people, and investing less time in high-technology answers."

"High-tech medicine is geared toward end-stage disease, not toward health care across the span of life."

"Health is more than sheer physical well-being. It has psychological and social underpinnings, and to understand these things is to help prevent sickness from happening. Family practitioners have more influence on health than any other doctors."

"The pediatrician is not going to be delirious about having a family practitioner come and do all the well-babies stuff. The internist is not going to be delirious about losing the once-a-month congestive heart failure or the diabetic who has to come in to have medications regulated. But about half of such specialists, interestingly enough, do support the family-practice movement. A couple of pediatricians here in town are delighted to have the family practitioners around, as long as they recognize a sick kid—a meningitis, a pneumonia not responding to antibiotics—and don't try to deal with that."

"I think people want to relate to somebody who can provide their health needs ninety per cent of the time and direct them to somebody else for the complex problems that are a one-shot thing."

"The family practitioner is not going to do colostomies and brain tumors or take out bleeding ulcers, but he sure is going to know when somebody may have those problems."

"There are certain kinds of problems where it's better not to be in the hands of a surgeon. Duodenal ulcer, for example, is not a surgical problem unless you bleed, perforate, obstruct. Certain kinds of thyroid problems don't need to be operated on. Those things can be followed by family practitioners. It is a fact of life that if a surgeon is two years out of training and has four children indications for operation are likely to be rather broad. If you're middle-aged, like me, and don't have kids to support in school, you can afford the luxury of total honesty and say to someone, 'You don't need an operation.' That's unfortunate, but to deny that it happens is crazy. The family practitioner keeps patients from falling into that kind of situation."

"Does this give us back our good family doctor? Of

course not! That would require re-creating the social context within which our family doctor was 'at home.' In an age where our medicine has attained such gigantic dimensions, any attempt in this direction can only spread us too thin, dilute our efforts, and lower our standards."

"If the old-time family doc had been meant to survive, he would have appropriately adapted in the evolution of American medicine."

"With remarkable perceptiveness, a hundred years ago, Dostoevsky satirically forecast the day when a medical specialist in problems of the right nostril would refer patients whose problem is on the left side."

"What the family practitioner is doing is routing people in the proper direction, finding the right person for the given diagnostic problem. Hiatus hernia is a good example, where there's a little relaxation and the stomach slides up into the chest and you may have a little heartburn. You can always find somebody who will operate on that. The family practitioner very quickly learns what surgeons will listen to that patient, treat him medically, and say he doesn't need an operation."

"They've got the right string but the wrong yo-yo. They are of the post-flower-child era—young people sincerely interested in being advocates for the patient and wanting to return to being complete physicians. They are well motivated but have only the artificial support of the society."

"I spend more time in the office listening to people than most surgeons do, because I like to know what's going on in their heads. If you have to take out their gallstones and you know their mother died after a gall-bladder operation, you can deal with it. If you don't know that, you just say, 'My dear, you have gallstones and we'll operate Tuesday.' If that patient doesn't do well, you don't know what the hell is going on. Many people tell me about problems they should have told their internist. I don't see the same thing happening when they've been to family practitioners. They're sympathetic, sensible—sort of a counsellor type, if you will. Internists are like the rest of us specialists. They want to do something about a problem and move on to the next one."

"Internists do what family practitioners do, but they only do it with adults. An oncologist does mostly oncology, true, but if you've got a cardiologist in a group of internists maybe thirty per cent of what he sees will be cardiology and thirty per cent of what the guy next to him sees will be cardiology, too. The difference is that within a group you maneuver and reallocate so that the more difficult cardiology patients wind up with the cardiologist. Same with gastroenterology. Everybody sees the same number of G.I. cases. It's just that the Crohn's disease and the ulcerative colitis will go to the gastro-enterologist. That is why internists say, 'What is family practice all about? We do that all the time. We do the same thing. We just don't take care of screaming, snotty-nosed kids.'"

"You can't have screaming children side by side with geriatric patients. You can't run an efficient office that way."

95

"You have an old man who's developing Alzheimer's disease. He is forgetful and spills peas on his shirt. You get a CAT scan and decide that Alzheimer's is the problem. You can then go on and on reconfirming the diagnosis. This is what happens when you get into the hands of a specialist. Next month, we get an electroencephalogram. Then we go to glucose tolerance to be sure we're not missing something—when all the patient needs is somebody to talk to."

"A person who's motivated to be with people in that way and who also knows when to tell you to go see a specialist—that's how it should work. That is the ideal of family practice. The only thing is: Can you take somebody who's in the top two per cent of intelligence in the United States and keep that person happy for forty years doing that?"

"Traditionally, the Harvard mission has been to train leaders in academic medicine. Leaders in academic medicine do not go to Presque Isle, Maine. In Amphitheatre E, at Harvard Medical School, our professors are always saying something like 'In this lecture hall sat Louis Diamond, who outlined the problem of Rh incompatibility between mother and child. One of you will one day make such a discovery, too.' They never say to us, 'One of you will go out and become the best doctor some little town ever had.' That is never said at Harvard Medical School, and never will be said. Harvard does not have a family-practice department. Once a year, there is a family-practice dinner, but the school provides little if any support. Despite the fact that the dean and the rest of the faculty do not like family practice, thirteen students from last year's class went on into family-practice residencies. An anomaly in Harvard's medical philosophy is that Harvard courses sometimes stress prevention, which is the particular province of family practice, and then they denigrate family practice. Roman DeSanctis, professor of medicine at Harvard and director of clinical cardiology at Massachusetts General—who has been celebrated as the physician of Henry Kissinger, the physician of John Wayne—gave a lecture about technological advances. As he ended, he said he would list the three most important things in cardiology: No. 1—prevention. No. 2—prevention. No. 3 —prevention. He said, 'Often, by the time these people get to me, there isn't all that much I can do for them.' That sort of thing is said in lectures—and at the same time they belittle the people who are out there doing the prevention."

"Canada has a lower death rate than we do, and broader medical care. Canada has doctors everywhere, in all the small towns. Sweden does, too. Meanwhile, we have all these high-tech doctors in cities with their machines. The United States is thirteenth on the life-expectancy list. Why is that? If we are doing things so right, how come we are thirteenth?"

Coming down the west side of Penobscot Bay and crossing the bridge over the mouth of the Passagassawakeag River, you see Belfast—red brick cubes spread up a hill above a harbor full of trawlers. By the water is a chicken factory and the marine terminus of the Belfast & Moosehead Lake Railroad, hauler of grain to feed the chickens. A road sign at the bridge says:

BELFAST
BROOKS
FREEDOM

At first glance, it appears to be some sort of pronouncement. Belfast is the home of Waldo County General Hospital, forty-nine beds, with a catchment of twenty-five thousand. This is where David Thanhauser—who still lives alone on his fifty acres six miles back from the sea—eventually decided to practice, after concluding that (in his words) "you don't have to be a superspecialist to do a good job." "Peyton Place" was filmed on location nearby—interesting milieu for a doctor trained in the health care of whole families. Among the people's occupational hazards are musculoskeletal and skin diseases that result from standing in one place doing the same thing all day long, such as yanking lungs out of chickens.

98

To an office on Northport Avenue, just behind the hospital, about twenty patients a day come to see this young doctor with his stethoscope draped around his neck like a collegiate scarf. He has full, thick, curly hair, an analgesic mustache, and he is likely to be wearing a button-down shirt (no tie), gray slacks, and Wallabees. Working alone, he moves from examining room to examining room, patient to waiting patient—and while waiting for him to appear virtually no one is shy to discuss him. "In order to treat a patient, it's vital to know the family environment," remarks Debbie Paradis, a large attractive tawny-haired woman who has come in with a hurting back that has been aggravated by her weight. Her husband, who is a pressman, and her son, Josh, are Thanhauser's patients, too. She was four when her parents died, and now says, "Sometimes I feel God cheated me. He took my parents young." She grew up a ward of the state, and, perhaps as a result, she speaks with a directness that has an ever-present cutting edge and no apparent guile. One believes her when she says of herself and Thanhauser, "We've batted heads a few times. But he's honest. That's why I know I can trust him. We felt a lot of doctors out before we picked David. He doesn't always tell you what you want. You call him, he's always there. He's been to our house more than once. I'm accident prone. All in the last four years, I stepped in a dog hole and broke my right foot, my appendix ruptured, I had Josh cesarean. David plays on a softball team. We love to walk by and watch him play. We feel he's almost one of the family. We know he's there for us when we need him. And not just for physical things. If you have a fight with your husband, he helps you try to understand that. Belfast is like Peyton Place. Do something when you're young, you have no second chance."

Man comes in with a cast on his leg and a maddening itch after five weeks. He has refrained from attempting to cut away the cast with his chain saw. "People do come in here who have tried to take off casts with chain saws," Thanhauser comments. Beneficially, such patients, while removing their casts, have thus far failed to remove their legs.

A young officer from a regional bank presents, as he has before, with a "pressure-type pain" in his chest.

"I continue to think that it's not your heart," Thanhauser tells him, attempting to treat the man's explicit fear. "Your discomfort disappears with food. On balance, it sounds like ulcer-type things. When you lie down, acid goes into the esophagus, causes heartburn—peptic-acid disease—and there is no burn in the stomach. That is classic. But if everything were classic this would be an easy job."

Lilly Greenleaf comes in with her husband, Lucky. She is a crab picker, nearing term, and he is an earth-science teacher. Indoors and out, he wears a five-gallon hat, and looks a good bit like a cowboy. "Some critter!" he says, listening through Thanhauser's stethoscope to the thundering heartbeats in Lilly's womb.

Lilly says, "From what I've read, the baby will have my allergies. It shares them with me in the womb."

"I don't know," Thanhauser replies. "I don't know how to answer that."

Routinely, he asks her if the baby will be under his care or if she will choose a pediatrician.

"Pediatrician," she says. "That's his specialty, isn't it?"

Amy Barden follows, carrying her three-month-old son, Rowen, who was born at home, with a midwife attending and a gathering of relatives present. Amy Barden is a robust woman of thirty with her hair in a bun. She began her day washing down the "parlor" in the family barn and doing what she calls calf chores—variously feeding her calves milk, hay, grain. The Bardens live twenty miles from Belfast, on three hundred and fifty acres. They have seventy milkers in their herd.

Thanhauser says he wants to give Rowen a D.P.T. shot. The P. stands for pertussis (whooping cough), the vaccine for which can cause a baby to become retarded. This happens to an extremely low percentage of babies. The vaccine, however, prevents whooping cough, which can also cause retardation—more frequently than the vaccine. Amy Barden refuses the D.P.T. Thanhauser reminds her that Maine law requires the shot and if she wishes to avoid it she must put her request in writing. He also says, "You are asking me to stick with an old medical philosophy, which is 'First, do no harm.' "

"Essentially, yes," says Amy Barden.

"Then maybe I'll get to see a case of whooping cough."

JOHN MCPHEE

"My mother had it, and she is alive to tell about it."

"Not everyone dies from whooping cough. In England, they stopped giving D.P.T. shots for a time, and discovered that more people were hurt by disease than had been by the shots."

Amy Barden listens politely and again refuses the shot.

People who refuse D.P.T. shots, polio drops, and the like depress Thanhauser. What depresses him, he remarks after she has gone, is not the refusal but the fact that the refusal makes him angry at his patient.

Waiting in an examining room is possibly the best-dressed baby in Maine, wearing a rose pastel dress and white leather shoes. The shoes keep her feet down. They tend to flex up. When she was born, Thanhauser sent her immediately to Portland, where a neurosurgeon did all he could to correct a spina bifida—a failure of fusion of posterior elements, which had left an opening between her central nervous system and her skin. Hydrocephalic as well, she underwent a shunt procedure, and now a tube is visible running beneath her skin from the top of her head to her abdomen. Her mother, an attractive woman in her early thirties, has in her appearance a suggestion of gauntness, a beleaguered look in her eyes. She and her husband and all three of her daughters are Dr. Thanhauser's patients. The family lives on a dirt road about a mile from the nearest telephone or commercial source of electric power. They built their house themselves, on eighty acres—a five-year project only recently completed. Now they will sell the place

102

and move to town. The baby has essentially no muscles in the backs of her legs, and will—at best—require braces to walk. Her eyesight has been affected, too, but might respond to surgery. There is nothing David Thanhauser can do for her in an ophthalmological or neurosurgical way, but he can do something no less beneficial. Between major medical events, he can watch, examine, explain. He can select referrals and guide the parents. He can be there when no one else would be.

Emily Hamilton, who is sixty-two, comes in with Einger West, who is eighty. Thanhauser prepares to give Einger West a flu shot. "He gives a good needle," Emily Hamilton says, in her voice the ring of promise.

"I'd like to put a little fat on your bones," Dr. Thanhauser says to Einger West, who replies, "I eat like a . . . like a . . ."

"Bird," Emily Hamilton says.

Einger West is wearing a bright-red pants suit, cream-colored clogs, and tinted glasses. Her husband died twenty years ago. She lives alone, and wants to go on living alone. Of all the things she might be persuaded to give up, the last would be her independence. Sometimes she has "spells." Her heart pounds, she feels as if she were "going away," the top of her head seems to be coming off, and she passes out. Thanhauser mentions hypoglycemia and adjustments in diet. He suggests Meals on Wheels.

"I can cook," Einger West snaps. "I can take care of myself."

Emily Hamilton says, "You have no muscles.

You're just skin hanging off your bones. That's all you are, Mama."

Einger West weighed a hundred and twenty-five pounds a few years ago; she now weighs ninety-two. Thanhauser asks her if she has given up smoking.

"Certainly not," she says.

"How much are you smoking?"

"A package a day. I take Vitamin C for the smoke."

"Alcohol?"

"I don't drink alcohol. You know that."

"How is your breathing these days?"

"It's all right. I walk to the mailbox. I can't hurry."

"May I have a look at those cataracts?"

"Oh, for heaven's sake, they don't bother me."

In the end, Thanhauser successfully insists on arranging for Meals on Wheels. And, as a final item, Emily Hamilton says, "Check her ears. She don't hear good."

"May I look in your ears?" Thanhauser says to Einger West.

And she says, "Yes, if you don't look too far."

Once a week, Thanhauser goes to Augusta and teaches in the residency of which he is a product. Occasionally, he sits in with residents as they see their patients—or, from another room (and with the patient's permission), watches them on closed-circuit television. Sometimes he videotapes a session, so that he and the resident can review it. If the resident uses terminology that the patient obviously does not understand, Thanhauser will remark on it, as he does if a resident gives a patient short shrift or, conversely, explores peripheral details to the point of wasting time. When a resident, full of programmed knowledge, delivers some sort of rehearsed recitation about the factors in a case while missing points and issues the patient would obviously like to raise, Thanhauser notes that, too. If a resident is made anxious by a patient's medical problem, the intimacy of television will reveal to Professor Thanhauser the resident's anxiety being transmitted to the patient. The residency has a faculty, full-time and part-time, approaching a hundred physicians. David Shinstrom and James Schneid, family practitioners, teach full time, as do Helen Mitchell, a pediatrician, and Daniel Onion, an internist. Frederic Craigie, Jr., Ph.D., is a full-time teacher of psychology. Paul Forman and Forrest West, from Albion, teach in the residency, too, as do Donna Conkling and Ann Dorney, from Skowhegan.

In late afternoon, residents and faculty collect around a conference table and review some of the items the day has brought and what was done about them— an aortic aneurysm, for example, and a spontaneous pneumothorax, and a sixteen-year-old who is both hypertensive and pregnant, and a fourteen-year-old who wanted contraceptive pills. Jargon flies about. "Technical virgins" have been the subjects of "curbside consultations" (a curbside consultation happens when one doctor stops another in the hall), and "emotional fire drills" are agreed to be as shrewdly precautionary as "engineering parents out of the room." Sometimes a topic vanishes into deep syntactical thickets: "She is sixteen and sexually active but only with one person at a time."

Residents in other specialties receive virtually no outpatient training. Even internists are expected—after leaving their residencies and entering practice—to pick up empirically the craft of dealing with the people who walk into their offices. Over three years, the Maine–Dartmouth residents spend about half their time in their own three-story Family Medicine Institute, in Augusta, high above the river and just across a parking lot from the Kennebec Valley Medical Center. The F.M.I., as it is known—with its multiple waiting rooms, laboratories, examining rooms, and television cameras—is something more than the educational conscience of the hospital across the way. Eight or ten residents hold office hours there on any given day, seeing nearly two thousand people a month who have learned that the young doctors in that brick building on East Chestnut Street are cheap, competent, and available—and prepared to take adequate time to explore a family history or explain as fully as possible the details of a disease. In ten years, the F.M.I. has metamorphosed the Kennebec Valley Medical Center from a community hospital into a teaching hospital—if not into a medical center. (The term "medical center" has spread to the most remarkable places— all in homage to urban-academic complexes like Beth Israel and Columbia Presbyterian, whose importance has created the resonance in the term. Little clapboard clinics in woods somewhere will call themselves medical centers, as do community hospitals in numerous cities and towns. Such widespread use of the term is no less legitimate than it is hubristic. The great teaching hospitals do not own those words. There would be no violation of fact if, up a trail in the Adirondacks, the owner of a log cabin were to call it the Empire State Building.) The Kennebec Valley hospital's quality as a congregation of working doctors has been elevated by the presence of the residency in part because, as a teaching hospital, it is a place where more questions are going to be asked than would be asked if the residency were not there. In teaching rounds, scheduled conferences, and other forms of interaction, the residents engender a running dialogue that tends to draw specialists together. While there is no way to quantify the effect of all this on the hospital— the summary enhancement of the level of patient care— it can be expressed anecdotally, and I am indebted to the residency's Alan Hume, vascular and general surgeon, for the following remarks and anecdotes: "A resident is always bugging you, asking things. If someone asks me a question and I don't know the answer, I come back tomorrow with an answer. This makes me a better doctor, and the patient gets better care. The resident is a built-in audit. . . . A resident is there when staff doctors are not. A first-year resident at the bedside is more valuable than a doctor on the telephone who has twenty years' experience. Even when the staff doctor is there, two heads are better than one. Suppose you've got a G.I.

bleeder admitted. You do X-ray studies. The resident suggests, 'Check the clotting mechanism. Maybe this patient has liver disease and isn't clotting properly.' Not infrequently, that's the problem. We all know that's one of the things you do, but—people being people, and not computers—you forget. Not long ago, an emergency situation came up—post-op on a ventilator, blood gases deteriorating. Patient getting a little confused. A resident suspected a spontaneous pneumothorax, and thought to stop the ventilator, get a good X-ray, and prove the diagnosis. He called me. I put a tube in the patient's chest to reexpand the lung. The thing turned right around. Without the resident, that would have been picked up twelve hours later, and the patient would not have done as well."

"Not done as well?"

"Not done as well. Which includes maybe not recovering. Residents quickly develop perceptions about who has the smarts in a given sphere. Ten per cent of any medical staff are not competent. They haven't kept up. The residency is at the heart of the continuing education of the medical staff. Ironically, some of the staff are not interested."

Looking back on her days in the F.M.I., Ann Dorney has remarked, "At the end of my second year, I felt I could handle anything. At the end of my third year, I was beginning to wonder." Early in the program, a family-practice resident develops a sense of the very wide range of patients who do not require attention that is beyond the competence of a family practitioner. In fact, roughly half the problems that are presented to a family doctor are not even organic in nature. Gradually and experientially, the residency also shows the new doctors their individual limitations. David Axelman has said, "One thing they're good at training you in is what you don't know. To be honest about it. Not to think you can do too much. Not to think you're a superman." In any field of medicine, doctors will vary not only in basic knowledge but also in manner, approach, and skill. In the words of Paul Forman, "Medical school is where you learn to be a doctor. The residency is where you learn what kind of doctor you are—where you mold your style. In family practice, the trick is knowing when to refer."

Referral is the fulcrum of the family practitioner's craft. From case to case—situation to situation, medical topic to medical topic—the exact position of the fulcrum varies with the doctor. One who too readily refers patients to assorted specialists is suffering a loss of science —giving up one chance after another to add experience in manageable situations. An ideal family practitioner works not just within but also up to the limits of her competence, his competence—knowing precisely where those limits are. Forman says, "You try to make the right scientific diagnosis with the least steps, try to make a good quick history that doesn't miss things. This is the real challenge of family practice. You know the health resources available to you. You don't hold on to patients too long out of pride or ignorance. The talent is in knowing when to give them up."

In some ways, a good family practitioner is not unlike a good bush pilot. There is no dearth of self-confident, highly skillful, bad bush pilots who cross the margins of heavy weather and whang into mountains. The good pilots know when to choose not to fly—know their own limitations and the limitations of their craft—and are unembarrassed by their decisions. "In the past year and a half, I have helped salvage six planes that were wrecked by *one* pilot," a very good bush pilot once said to me. "Why do passengers *go* with such pilots? Would they go to the moon with an astronaut who did not have round-trip fuel? If you were in San Francisco and the boat to Maui was leaking and the rats were leaving, even if you had a ticket you *would not go*. Safety in the air is where you find it. Proper navigation helps, but proper judgment takes care of all conditions. You say to yourself, 'I ain't going to go today. The situation is too much for me.' And you resist all pressure to the contrary."

When outpatients appear in the F.M.I. with problems that are beyond the competence of the residents, they are routinely referred to specialists and subspecialists on the staffs of Kennebec Valley and other hospitals. They can be referred up the system to Portland and beyond. When something perplexing suggests neurology, however, the residents can step to an intercom and call upstairs, asking for their director, Alexander McPhedran.

Here, for example, Tim Clifford, a second-year resident, sees a patient whose name is Elaine Ladd. She is twenty-two years old, small, slim, light on her feet, with uncorrected teeth, a sweeping and engaging smile. She wears a print dress. Her blond hair is gathered in a band. She reports what Clifford records as a six-month history of right-leg weakness. As she got out of bed one day, she fell to the floor. Another day, she fell, unaccountably, on a flight of stairs. There have been similar occasions, in all of which, when the leg collapsed, the knee did not buckle. At these times, her right foot and leg felt heavy, her toes tingled, and the sole of her right foot was numb. She has had some pain but has taken no medicines. She has minor curvature of the spine, Clifford notes. Three years ago, when she was nineteen, she gave birth to a baby—experiencing a normal delivery—and now this pretty and curly-haired child runs in the F.M.I. hallway and bounces in and out of the examining room while Tim Clifford examines her mother. The cranial nerves are intact. There is no arm drift. Her gait is normal. Her biceps and triceps are normal. Clifford excuses himself and, with the help of the intercom and the magic of beeperology, asks Alex McPhedran to join him. The two doctors meet in the first-floor hallway. Clifford says he can find nothing to suggest a problem. If it were not for the stories of the patient's repeated falling, he would call her absolutely normal.

McPhedran follows Clifford into the examining room and, with Elaine Ladd, is soon in a dialogue much encircled by her child.

"Three times I have fallen—once when I got up to chase my daughter."

"Do you exercise regularly?"

"No. I just walk."

"When you walk, how far do you go?"

"Ten miles."

"Does the tingling go away as you walk?"

"Yes."

"This has been going on for six months?"

"Yes."

"Why are you here now?"

"I'm scared. I'm scared when I have no feeling in my toes. I've never told this to anyone before: I paint. Sometimes, when I am doing something very delicate, my hand shakes. Also, I faint."

"Frequently?"

"Yes."

"Does your hand shake at other times—for example, when you are putting a pin in a diaper?"

Elaine Ladd contemplates Dr. McPhedran. Her look is quizzical. "A pin?" she says.

"Oh," says McPhedran, perceptibly taken aback. "I guess I am showing my age. People don't put pins in diapers anymore. Sorry about that."

McPhedran, in his fifties, is a large-framed, pleasant man with a long toss of hair, a bemused smile, and a look which suggests, correctly, that he rises early, works late, and worries on Sunday. He asks to see Elaine Ladd's back and, with a broad-nibbed pen, draws a line down her spine. He says, "Is there someone who can clean this off for you?"

"No," she answers. "But I have a back-scrubber."

A nurse comes into the room and hands McPhedran a slip of paper. He looks at it and learns of the birth of his first grandchild. He sets aside his reactions, making no remark. He opens a safety pin and asks Elaine Ladd to say, as he presses it against this and that place on her feet and lower legs, whether the sensation is dull or sharp. In random choice, he turns the pin, as she says, "Dull, shop . . . Dull, shop . . . Shop, shop, dull, dull, shop."

He breaks a tongue depressor to obtain a short sharp stick, and with considerable pressure he scrapes the stick across the soles of her feet. "I'm sorry," he says. "I know it's sort of irritating."

She tells him not to be concerned.

When he scrapes the bottom of her right foot, her toes do not go down.

Soon McPhedran and Clifford withdraw to a porch at one end of the F.M.I. In the course of their conversation, McPhedran explores the case rhetorically, asking himself questions: "Is it in a peripheral nerve? Is it a cord lesion?"

And Clifford tells him, "I see no way to go further without involving her in your thinking."

McPhedran, for the moment, continues to think aloud. He says, "You can test sensory-evoked potentials without hurting the patient at all. This is what the space age has done for neurological physiology."

Clifford says, "I think the patient should hear right away what someone thinks. She can't just go home and sit around."

McPhedran agrees, but, returning to the examining room, follows his intuition. He mentions a lumbar puncture—a spinal tap—and tests of the eyes he would like her to have. "It's a good idea to find out about it," he goes on. "You wouldn't have come in if it weren't a nuisance. And I think we ought to pursue it."

Elaine Ladd meets his gaze brightly, agreeably, and seems not to be dissatisfied with the quantity of what he is saying. She frames no question. He has edged up to and around his thoughts, which, for the time being, he elects to keep to himself. This could be a meningioma of the spinal cord. He does not think so. It could be scoliosis—progressing, and affecting the nervous system. He does not think so. He thinks her problem is multiple sclerosis.

McPhedran is in many ways a walking microcosm of the family-practice movement, a man whose professional career is a CAT scan of the medicine of his time. He grew up in the Germantown section of Philadelphia, the son of a specialist in pulmonary diseases, and was educated at Harvard College and Harvard Medical School. As a medical student, he was interested principally in developing general competence, so he gravitated toward internal medicine. Even more, he was drawn to doing clinical teaching in a big city—this because he admired his teachers and the role they were playing in the medical system. The most interesting teachers, he thought, were the neurologists, probably because so much of what they did depended on interviewing, examining—activities that framed the whole patient. Under the influence of these academic neurologists, his interests gradually narrowed and deepened. Following two years of residency in internal medicine at Beth Israel in Boston, he added three years in neurology at Massachusetts General and one year in Harvard Medical School's laboratory of neurophysiology. Ready to teach, he was hired by Emory University, in Atlanta, as, in his words, "their neurophysiology person." He taught there for ten years. He taught medical residents, neurosurgical residents, and neurologists, meanwhile concentrating his own special interest ever more exclusively on electromyography—the study of electrical activity in muscles. As a member of the Department of Medicine, he was an attending physician on the medical floor; nonetheless, as he became increasingly subspecialized in neurology he saw a diminishing variety of patients. "Gradually, you get to know more and more about less and less," he comments. "Eventually, I realized that I could not even manage a person with hypertension. There were many medical problems I knew nothing about. I felt a slipping, or lost, competency in general medicine. Even in neurology, my competency was narrowing. I did no pediatric neurology, for example. I felt my general competence slipping away while I became ever more adept with oscilloscopes and amplifiers, measuring the electrical activity of nerves and muscles, diagnosing neuromuscular diseases or establishing that the nerves and muscles were healthy. An electromyographer has no patients of his own. An electromyographer does tests for someone else. On the economic side of it, the sad fact is that people who want to make a high income in medicine learn to do things like electromyography. More than science attracts people to such fields. In Maine, the present cost for an electromyogram is two hundred and forty dollars. The procedure takes about as long as a complete physical exam and costs at least three times as much. The money in medicine these days is in tests and procedures, and this leads to conflicts of interest—to tests that are not necessary. To be part of the system, an electromyographer does not say that an electromyogram is unnecessary and refuse to do one. Patients, for their part, never protest charges for tests. The public seems to value tests and procedures to an extent that is not justified by their relative scientific value. Good clinical judgment is more important than tests."

As doctors in increasing numbers went into tests and procedures, their vernacular changed, too, and they began to chat intensely about the "marketing of services." The phrase did not rest comfortably on Celtic sensibilities. When McPhedran heard metropolitan-hospital doctors saying things like "How can we market our services to the people upcountry so that they will send us patients?" he wondered who might actually be out there seeing the patients upcountry.

McPhedran was appointed to the National Advisory Council for Regional Medical Programs, went to Washington regularly, and made site visits all over the United States. On these journeys, what he discerned most immediately was that primary-care physicians were disappearing. He visited regions where there were no physicians at all. Elsewhere, everybody was a "consul-tant." Almost everyone was in a city, running tests. "In many places, there were specialists, but no one was responsible for continuing care of patients. While the O.B.–G.Y.N.s were taking care of women's procreative organs, many patients were without a regular doctor. Internists were doing it. But they were not around in sufficient numbers to take care of everyone. Also, they did just adults."

Back home, he often found himself asking some-one, "Who is your doctor?"

The person would say something like "I had a doc-tor, but he moved away. Can you take care of me?"

And McPhedran would say, "No. I'm a consultant in neurology at the Emory Clinic."

On one of his federal assignments, he happened into Maine—a state with no medical school and a scarcity of rural doctors, a state attempting to set up a family-practice residency that would siphon new doctors out of the megalopolis and sprinkle them through the northern countryside. By teaching in such a residency, he decided, he could help train physicians for primary care, continue to do neurology, and possibly regain the medical perspective he felt that he had lost. In his strong reaction to the increased subspecialization of his own career, he gave up university teaching, abandoned the developing subtleties of electromyography, moved to Maine, and soon began preparing for family-practice board examinations. When he took them and passed, he became a family practitioner. Not a few people were saying that family practice was a fad. McPhedran saw it as a trend—a change in the profession's view of itself.

McPhedran's manner amuses his students, who regard his politeness as bordering on the eccentric—a man who apologizes to patients for scratching the bottoms of their feet, who says to patients, almost apologetically, "Did I answer your question? Did I tell you what you wanted? I'm grateful to you for asking questions. I'd rather have you ask them than go away wondering." For all his super-subspecialized neurological skills, he is the quintessential family doctor, listening closely, empathetic—out of the basements of neurology, into the world. To be sure, he still spends a good deal of time reading electroencephalograms, and not a little reading music.

For the F.M.I.'s standard twenty-five-dollar office-visit fee, Alexander McPhedran now spends forty-five minutes with a woman who will leave him feeling as if he had been with her all day. The gulf between them is wide indeed. She wants—insists upon—neurosurgery. He suggests that she try Anacin instead. The neurologist in him knows that surgery is contraindicated for her type of facial pain. The neurologist could say that and be done with it. As a family practitioner, though, he will try to deal with the pain—and with a mind that is set in the direction of a surgical fix.

"When I go to a doctor, I expect to be given something, and I expect it to work," she says. "If I need surgery, I expect to have surgery. I have had this pain for two months, and I want it over with."

McPhedran tells her in a flat voice that no reputable neurosurgeon would operate on her. She looks doubtful. She says she will check that out. McPhedran admits the possibility that Anacin might fail her. In that eventuality, he says, he recommends Excedrin. After she leaves, he remarks, "The placebo effect of surgery is high. A sham operation might do it for her. But I have to protect her from such a procedure if I can."

Amy Hufnagel comes in, breezily says "Hi" to Dr. McPhedran, tells him she is a bit pressed to be on time for a field-hockey game, and sticks out her tongue. Amy Hufnagel is a robust, athletic, attractive teen-ager with long brunette hair, an overt sense of humor, and an ability to score goals. She wears a tartan shirt, a green corduroy skirt. There are two pearls in each ear. About her tongue she is not at all self-conscious. In the corridors of Winthrop High School, she enjoys cornering some unsuspecting friend and saying, "Look! Do you want to see something gross?" With which she sticks out her tongue. It is wrinkled up like a calf's brain. It has a caved-in side. It twitches. As she sticks it out now for McPhedran, a large part of the surface, on the left side, leaps and bubbles like boiling soup. A part of it has atrophied as well—a baylike indentation. The tongue dances. It humps. Amy laughs. Her speech is not affected. She has difficulty eating some foods but no additional inconvenience. McPhedran tests—as he has on other occasions—the nerves and muscles of her mouth, face, and eyes. All are normal. The pharynx nerve is normal. In recent months, there has been some clicking in her left ear. He has no idea what to make of that. He does not know what to make of the whole situation. She has been his patient for more than a year. He calls her condition hemiatrophy of the tongue, but that is merely a description. Something is apparently going on in the twelfth nerve on the left side, but he cannot say what it is. Could it be mononeuropathy multiplex? In nearly thirty years in neurology, he has not seen the like of it.

When to refer. If a capacity for making that decision is the supreme talent of the family practitioner, it is no less relevant from time to time in the experience of a subspecialist. This neurologist—of course—has long since referred this patient to higher authority. When McPhedran comes upon something that is beyond his range, his reading, his neurological comprehension, he sends the patient to his own incomparable mentor—Raymond D. Adams, of Harvard University and Massachusetts General Hospital, a master of clinical analysis. Adams is unfailingly accommodating. He knows he will see something interesting if it comes from Alex.

Amy, her mother, and her father went to Boston. They spent two days there and returned to Augusta. Afterward, Raymond D. Adams wrote to Alexander McPhedran, "The Hufnagels are a delightful family." That was the extent of his diagnosis. He had absolutely no idea what was wrong with Amy's tongue.